# Occupational Therapy and Duchenne Muscular Dystrophy

D0841905

## DATE DUE

| | |
|---|---|
| MAR 1 8 2008 | |
| JUL 0 5 2017 ~~FEB 2 7 2012~~ | |
| AUG 0 2 2017 | |
| | |
| | |
| | |
| | |
| | |
| | |
| | |
| | |
| | |
| | |

# Occupational Therapy and Duchenne Muscular Dystrophy

By
KATE STONE, CLAIRE TESTER, ALEX HOWARTH,
RUTH JOHNSTON, NICOLA TRAYNOR,
HEATHER McANDREW, JOY BLAKENEY
AND MARY MCCUTCHEON

John Wiley & Sons Ltd

*Other Wiley Editorial Offices*

John Wiley & Sons Inc., 111 River Street, Hoboken, NJ 07030, USA

Jossey-Bass, 989 Market Street, San Francisco, CA 94103-1741, USA

Wiley-VCH Verlag GmbH, Boschstr. 12, D-69469 Weinheim, Germany

John Wiley & Sons Australia Ltd, 42 McDougall Street, Milton, Queensland 4064, Australia

John Wiley & Sons (Asia) Pte Ltd, 2 Clementi Loop #02-01, Jin Xing Distripark, Singapore
129809

John Wiley & Sons Canada Ltd, 6045 Freemont Blvd, Mississauga, ONT, L5R 4J3

Wiley also publishes its books in a variety of electronic formats. Some content that appears in
print may not be available in electronic books.

Anniversary Logo Design: Richard J. Pacifico

*Library of Congress Cataloging-in-Publication Data*

Occupational therapy and Duchenne muscular dystrophy / by Kate Stone . . . [et al.].
    p.  ;  cm.
    Includes bibliographical references and index.
    ISBN 978-0-470-51030-8 (alk. paper)
    1. Duchenne muscular dystrophy – Treatment.    2. Duchenne muscular dystrophy – Patients –
Rehabilitation.    3. Occupational therapy for children.    I. Stone, Kate.
    [DNLM:  1. Muscular Dystrophy, Duchenne–psychology–Case Reports.    2. Muscular
Dystrophy, Duchenne – therapy – Case Reports.    3. Occupational Therapy – methods –
Case Reports.    4. Quality of Life – Case Reports.    WE 559 O15 2007]
    RJ482.D78O33 2007
    616.7'4806 – dc22

                                                                              2007011293

*A catalogue record for this book is available from the British Library*

ISBN 13: 978-0-470-51030-8

Typeset by SNP Best-set Typesetter Ltd., Hong Kong
Printed and bound in Great Britain by TJ International Ltd, Padstow, Cornwall

This book is printed on acid-free paper responsibly manufactured from sustainable forestry in
which at least two trees are planted for each one used for paper production.

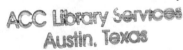

# Contents

# Contributors

*Joy Blakeney*, Dip COT, Senior Practitioner, Paediatric Community Occupational Therapist, formerly of West Lothian Council Social Work Department.

*Alex Howarth*, BSc Occupational Therapy, Senior Paediatric Occupational Therapist, NHS Lothian University Hospitals Division.

*Ruth Johnston*, BSc (Hons) Occupational Therapy, Senior Occupational Therapist – Child Health, NHS Fife.

*Heather McAndrew*, BSc (Hons) Occupational Therapy, Senior Paediatric Occupational Therapist, NHS Borders.

*Mary McCutcheon*, Dip COT, Senior Paediatric Occupational Therapist, formerly of Ashcraig School, Glasgow.

*Kate Stone*, Dip COT, MSc (MedSci) in Palliative Care, Senior Practitioner, Paediatric Community Occupational Therapist, Inverclyde Council Social Work Services.

*Claire Tester*, Dip COT, PG Dip, AHP Consultant in Cancer for Scotland, Scottish Executive on secondment from the Children's Hospice Association, Scotland (CHAS).

*Nicola Traynor*, BSc Occupational Therapy, Senior Paediatric Occupational Therapist, NHS Lothian University Hospitals Division.

# Preface

This book has been produced by core members of the Scottish Occupational Therapy Focus group for Muscular Dystrophy. Based on the authors' knowledge and experience, the intention is to provide a resource that facilitates a flexible and informed clinical approach to occupational therapy with this client group.

# Acknowledgements

We are very grateful to:
Dr Alison Wilcox, Clinical Coordinator, Scottish Muscle Network, Duncan Guthrie Institute of Medical Genetics, Yorkhill Hospitals, Glasgow for her assistance with the Medical Overview chapter and her contribution to the final chapter. We are also grateful to all the families affected by Duchenne muscular dystrophy who have shared their experiences with the therapists.

Acknowledgement and thanks are extended to the families and staff at Rachel House Children's Hospice, Kinross, Scotland and staff at children's hospices in the U.K. Especial thanks to Clare Watson, Jackie Armour, Paul McGinley and Daniel Morrison.

Acknowledgements and thanks to Angela Millar, Lesley Wotherspoon and Pat Carragher.

Acknowledgement and thanks are given to the managers and colleagues who have supported the therapists in completing this work. The relevant employers are:

- Inverclyde Council Social Work Services, Inverclyde Centre for Independent Living, Greenock.
- NHS Borders.
- NHS Fife.
- NHS Lothian University Hospitals Division.
- West Lothian Council Social Work Department.

The authors would especially like to thank their own families and friends for their support and patience.

# 1 Duchenne Muscular Dystrophy: A Medical Overview

**ALEX HOWARTH**

Duchenne muscular dystrophy is the most common and usually most severe form of muscular dystrophy (Kapsa et al., 2003). It is named after Dr Duchenne de Boulogne – a mid-nineteenth-century French physician, who was one of the first people to study and document some of the muscular dystrophies.

Duchenne muscular dystrophy is an X-linked recessive muscle-wasting disorder, involving progressive muscle weakness which normally becomes evident before the age of five years in an affected boy. A defective gene on the X chromosome (at Xp21 site) leads to a deficiency in dystrophin – a rod-shaped cytoskeletal protein which normally maintains the integrity of the muscle cell wall. Where dystrophin is deficient, there is an influx of calcium ions, a breakdown of the calcium calmodulin complex and an excess of free radicals. These changes lead eventually to irreversible destruction of the muscle cells. Dystrophin is also found in the brain and its deficiency is associated with cognitive impairment to a varying degree (Anderson et al., 2002; Leet et al., 2002).

In X-linked recessive inheritance, it is generally the males that are affected because the mutated allele on the X chromosome is not balanced by a normal allele, as it is in the case of females (males have X and Y chromosomes, whereas females have two X chromosomes). In approximately half to two-thirds of all cases of Duchenne muscular dystrophy, the mother carries the defective gene. In these cases, the female relatives of the carrier mother should be offered genetic counselling. The remaining cases arise through spontaneous mutation and, in these instances, female relatives will have the normal population risk of having an affected male child. For the general population, the risk of having an affected child is one in every 3,500–4,000 male births (Lissauer & Claydon, 1997; Nowak & Davies, 2004).

Female carriers are usually healthy, although a small number have a mild degree of weakness themselves and are then known as manifesting carriers. Daughters of affected males will all be carriers, whilst sons will not be affected, since a man passes a Y chromosome to his son. Each son of a female carrier has a 50% risk of being affected, and each daughter a 50% risk of being a carrier.

There are around 1,500 boys with Duchenne muscular dystrophy living in the UK at any one time. About 100 are born with the condition each year. Diagnosis is often made on clinical grounds supported by laboratory tests. The serum creatine phosphokinase is normally grossly elevated (normal values are in the lower hundreds, depending on the particular laboratory, but, in Duchenne muscular dystrophy, this figure will be in the high thousands). At this stage, a blood sample would also be sent to the genetics laboratory to look for a deletion or duplication on the X chromosome. If no deletion or duplication is identified, the next stage would be to proceed to a muscle biopsy. An absence of dystrophin staining on immunocytochemical staining together with the other changes typical of Duchenne muscular dystrophy, such as variation in muscle fibre size, muscle fibre necrosis, regeneration and replacement by fat, would confirm the diagnosis of Duchenne muscular dystrophy.

Once a mutation has been identified in a family, the female relative should be offered genetic counselling. Identification of carrier females requires interpretation of pedigree and specific tests: 70% of carrier females have a raised creatine phosphokinase level. Accurate carrier and prenatal diagnosis can also be made through DNA testing for gene deletion, duplication or point mutation. In the case in which a mutation has been identified in the affected male but not in the mother, there is a chance that the mutation has arisen in the ovaries of the mother. This is called Gonadal Mosaicism. However, tests for this are not available at the present time. In these cases, there is a 5% risk of having a further affected male child. Prenatal diagnosis should therefore be offered to these women.

## CLINICAL FEATURES

Symptoms usually begin between the second and sixth year of life (Rogers et al., 2001). The average age of diagnosis is 5.5 years, although children are usually referred for a medical opinion when much younger. Involvement begins in the proximal musculature of the pelvic girdle, proceeds to the shoulder girdle and finally affects all muscle groups, including the respiratory and heart muscles. Gower's Sign, in which the child uses his arms to crawl up his thighs into a standing position from a kneeling position, is diagnostically significant. Other indicators include: delayed walking; a waddling gait; toe-walking; a reluctance to walk; difficulty rising from a sitting or lying position; an inability to hop, skip or jump; frequent falling and stumbling; problems climbing stairs and running; cramp in the legs; and excessive fatigue. Enlargement of the calf, and sometimes of the forearm and thigh, is also characteristic. It is known as *pseudo*-hypertrophy because the enlargement of the muscle is not due to additional muscle fibres, but to replacement of the muscle fibres by fat and fibrous tissue. Progressive atrophy and weakness lead boys to become wheelchair-dependent, usually at between eight and eleven years of age. Joint contractures at the hip, knee and ankle and spinal deformities (scoliosis, kyphosis and lordosis) are common complications.

Duchenne muscular dystrophy is a life-limiting condition but, with improvement in management in areas such as the introduction of steroids (while the boys are still ambulant), postural management (once they are wheelchair-bound), spinal-fusion surgery, non-invasive ventilation and possibly more intense cardiac surveillance and management, the prognosis is improving. At present, many patients will die as a result of cardiac or respiratory failure (Eagle et al., 2002). Without ventilatory support, the average age of death is around 19 years but, where cardiac and respiratory functions are effectively managed, a survival to the third or fourth decade is not unknown (Brown, 2002; Bushby et al., 2005; Simonds, 2001).

Respiratory management is a subject that needs to be approached with sensitivity. In some cases, discussion of overnight ventilation may lead the family to appreciate fully for the first time that Duchenne muscular dystrophy is a life-limiting condition. Strong emotive reactions to this form of intervention may then ensue – total rejection on the one hand, an exaggerated sense of dependency on the other. In general, medical information may have to be explained several times to allow the families to absorb it fully and make fully informed decisions about future options.

## KEY POINTS

• Duchenne muscular dystrophy is the most common and usually most severe form of muscular dystrophy. It is a life-limiting condition.
• It is an X-linked recessive muscle-wasting disorder leading to a deficiency in dystrophin – a protein which normally protects the integrity of the muscle cell wall. Dystrophin is also found in the brain and its deficiency is associated with cognitive impairment.
• In X-linked recessive inheritance, it is generally the males that are affected. In approximately half to two-thirds of all cases, the mother carries the defective gene. Spontaneous mutation is responsible for the rest.
• Daughters of affected males will be carriers; each son of a female carrier has a 50% risk of being affected, and each daughter a 50% risk of being a carrier.
• About 1,500 boys are affected with Duchenne muscular dystrophy in the UK at any one time. About 100 are born with the condition every year.
• Diagnosis is often made on clinical grounds supported by laboratory tests. The serum creatine phosphokinase is usually grossly elevated. Duplication or deletion on the X chromosome would then be investigated through blood sampling. Muscle biopsy would be carried out if no deletion or duplication is found. An absence of dystrophin, variation in muscle fibre size, muscle

fibre necrosis, regeneration and replacement by fat would confirm a diagnosis of Duchenne muscular dystrophy.

- Accurate carrier and prenatal diagnosis can be made through DNA testing for gene depletion, duplication or point mutation.
- Symptoms usually begin between the second and sixth years of life. The average age of diagnosis is 5.5 years and wheelchair dependency occurs at between eight and eleven years.
- Involvement begins in proximal musculature of the pelvic girdle, proceeds to the shoulder girdle and finally affects all muscle groups, including the respiratory and heart muscles.
- The Gower's Sign (a characteristic method of transferring from kneeling to standing) is diagnostically significant. Delayed walking, a waddling gait, problems with stairs and running, leg cramps, excessive fatigue and pseudo-hypertrophy are other indicators.
- Prognosis is improving through developments in respiratory and cardiac management, the introduction of steroids, postural management and spinal-fusion surgery.

# 2 The Occupational Therapy Process

**KATE STONE, WITH CLAIRE TESTER**
**AND MARY McCUTCHEON**

## INTRODUCTION

Occupational therapists have a unique role in supporting and working with young men with Duchenne muscular dystrophy and their families, as they can assess and evaluate an individual's physical, psychological and social needs.

The occupational therapist's focus is on maximising skills, promoting and enabling independence, as well as improving the quality of life of the family. It follows that occupational therapists normally have an ongoing role in the treatment of young men with Duchenne muscular dystrophy.

Individuals will have contact with many occupational therapists and they may have more than one occupational therapist at a time involved in their care. Occupational therapists can be employed by a number of different agencies, with each agency being responsible for providing different services. This can cause confusion for some families, so it is extremely important that they have a clear understanding of each occupational therapist's role.

The vast majority of parents and children, when they first encounter an occupational therapist, are usually not sure of the occupational therapist's function. They normally associate the occupational therapist with the issue that has brought them to the house, such as 'it's the woman about the bath' or 'the man that deals with the boy's handwriting'. Both of these are a small aspect of the services that an occupational therapist can provide and, therefore, each occupational therapist involved with the family needs to clarify what services their agency can offer.

Where there is good communication and cooperation between the different occupational therapy services, they can often offer better services than each individual service can provide.

This chapter defines occupational therapy and provides an overview of the skills that a therapist can offer when working with an individual with Duchenne muscular dystrophy.

## DEFINITION OF OCCUPATIONAL THERAPY

Occupational therapy is a health profession concerned with promoting health and well-being through occupation. Occupation in this sense means the activities that people have to do in their everyday life, such as personal-care tasks, like eating or bathing. It also includes other occupations, like housework, play, schoolwork and employment tasks. Occupational therapists work with people who have health problems to enable them to be as independent as possible in carrying out these occupations by helping them to regain their skills or by offering them alternative ways of participating in activities to improve their quality of life.

According to Blom-Cooper (1989, p. 14), the public and other professionals can have false and damaging stereotypes of the functions of occupational therapy and he recommended defining occupational therapy as follows:

'Occupational therapy is the assessment and treatment in conjunction and collaboration with other professional workers in health and social services, of people of all ages with physical and mental health problems, through specifically selected and graded activities, in order to help them reach their maximum level of functioning and independence in all aspects of daily life, which includes their personal independence, employment, social, recreational and leisure pursuits and their inter-personal relationships.'

This definition was created in the era before community care and does not include the educational aspects of the occupational therapy profession. A recent study by Creek (2006) looked at 37 different definitions of occupational therapy, with a view to creating one definitive definition; they did not succeed in this task, which is not surprising when one considers all the different elements of occupational therapy.

The philosophy of occupational therapy states that occupation is central to normal human existence and that its absence is a threat to health. It also holds that all individuals are of value and are inherently different and that a therapist must work with the individual to select meaningful activities to maintain personal well-being in a relevant social and cultural setting (Turner et al., 2002).

Occupational therapists work with all age groups in many different settings. Health boards or local authorities and government agencies can employ them, as can voluntary organisations and charities. Others work in housing agencies and education authorities, and some are in private practice. There are also occupational therapists working in universities and for commercial companies. Appendix I illustrates the basic knowledge base of occupational therapists.

The settings in which occupational therapists work are numerous and the following is a list of the main areas in which people with Duchenne muscular dystrophy may cross paths with occupational therapists:

- hospitals and clinics;
- wheelchair services;
- schools and nurseries;
- disabled-living centres;
- social work offices;
- housing agencies;
- hospices;
- equipment suppliers;
- charity organisations like the Muscular Dystrophy Campaign;
- job centres;
- in their own home.

Occupational therapy is a process of assessment, planning, intervention and evaluation. This is a continual process with people with Duchenne muscular dystrophy, as their needs and the needs of their carers are constantly changing.

In order for treatment to be effective, occupational therapists have to work closely with the family and other professionals involved with the family to ensure that treatment goals are realistic and achievable. Treatment is more effective if a proper assessment of the issues is carried out.

## ASSESSMENT

The main goal of assessment in occupational therapy is to get a clear understanding of the individual, their social circumstances and their environment, in order to develop a treatment plan which will improve the quality of life of the person and their family. The quality of the assessment carried out will have a direct correlation with the quality of the treatment interventions (Turner et al., 2002).

Ideally, in the atmosphere of evidence-based practice, standardised assessments should be used to measure the effectiveness of occupational therapy interventions. A standardised assessment is one which has been administered to a selected population and standard scores have been obtained that can be used to set a scoring procedure. The test is usually administered in a set way and the person being assessed is measured against the standardised sample to identify their level of performance.

At the time of writing, there are no standardised occupational therapy assessment tools that are specific to people with Duchenne muscular dystrophy. Occupational therapists and other professionals have created many standardised tests that could be used to assess certain functions that are problematic for people with Duchenne muscular dystrophy, but, if another professional has created the assessment, their objectives for testing may be entirely different from an occupational therapist's. This should be considered when selecting standardised assessments.

There are many standardised assessments that can be used to measure specific issues, such as handwriting, activities of daily living and cognitive assessments, etc. Due to the variety and number of these assessments, it is not possible to cover these within this chapter. However, the following reports (Edmans et al., 2001) include some considerations that should be taken into account when selecting standardised assessments which may be useful:

- What client group was the test designed for?
- How valid and reliable is the test?
- Is it validated for an occupational therapist to administer?
- How easy is the test to use?
- How long does it take to complete the test?
- Will an individual with Duchenne muscular dystrophy have the stamina, functional ability and concentration to complete the test?
- Is it age-appropriate for the individual?
- Is the issue important enough for the individual to warrant very detailed assessment?

Assessments are used to identify problems and how these problems are affecting the lifestyle of the individual and the family. They are also a basis for deciding whether occupational therapy interventions will be of assistance to the family.

The following are the main issues that Leeson (1995) recommends assessing for a child with special needs. These areas of assessment are equally relevant for a child with Duchenne muscular dystrophy. Additional areas need to be assessed with young adults and each individual will have other issues that may require assessment.

EXPECTATIONS

The first issue that an occupational therapist has to assess is what the family expects from their service. They may have made a simple request for information regarding equipment, etc. and may only wish to have that information supplied without further assessment or treatment. The occupational therapist's first assessment will be to decide the level of assessment that is required for each referral. That being said, the occupational therapist should inform the family of interventions that are available from their service. This could be in the form of a simple leaflet.

The occupational therapist then has to establish what issues are important for the family so that the initial assessments and treatments focus on the problems that are causing the most anxiety to the family. When and where the assessments are carried out also needs to be clarified.

## SOCIAL CIRCUMSTANCES

The social circumstances, work and lifestyle of a family have to be taken into account, as they can have a direct bearing on the occupational therapy interventions that can be offered. An assessment of the family's social situation may also indicate that there is a need for services other than occupational therapy.

## FAMILY COMPOSITION AND RELATIONSHIPS

The therapist also has to understand the composition and relationships within the family, as these will give some insight into the work and care demands made on each member of the family. The family's social network can also give an indication of the amount of informal support that the family may be able to access. It may also reveal how isolated the family is from the rest of society.

## CARE ARRANGEMENTS

Details should be collected regarding all the formal care support that is provided and when it is offered. This can be care provided at home, day care or residential care away from home. It is also necessary to check whether the care provided is meeting the needs of the family.

## EMOTIONAL SUPPORT FOR THE CHILD AND FAMILY

The therapist needs to ascertain the family members' understanding and attitude to the person's condition. There are many stages in the course of this illness during which the individual and the family are under a great deal of emotional stress. In addition, other issues can occur and these can cause great turmoil within a family. How the family copes with these issues should be considered but to assess this type of issue takes time and it is necessary for the occupational therapist to have established a good relationship with the family and the individuals within it before they will have a clear picture of how they are coping. It can be very obvious that someone is very distressed on a first visit and positive actions should be taken to try and reduce the person's stress levels.

## FINANCIAL SITUATION

As there may be charges for some services, the family's financial situation should be clarified to make sure that they are getting all their benefit entitlements and to check whether they will be liable for any charges for services.

## HOUSING

Housing is a major issue for people with muscular dystrophy. Most houses will have to be adapted to accommodate such a person, so a detailed assessment of the house is necessary to determine what housing adaptations are required and whether they can be carried out. When the house cannot be adapted to meet the needs of the family or the house is too small for the family, an assessment of their housing needs should be completed.

## MEDICAL

Information on the type of medication used is required and particulars of any previous or planned surgery are crucial, especially if the person has had their spine fused. It is also important to know whether ventilation is planned or used. Determine whether the individual is having sleeping problems. Details of any other medical conditions should also be recorded. If the child has learning difficulties or cognitive problems, this should be noted. If the individual is in pain, try to establish the cause of the pain. The medical conditions of other members of the family should also be documented.

## MOBILITY

A full evaluation of the person's mobility has to be undertaken to ensure that any mobility equipment that is being used still meets the needs of the individual. This assessment should include fall risks for an individual who is still walking and standing between transfers. Mobility within the bed and while seated should also be checked to make sure that the person can relieve pressure. The person's ability to walk over distance should also be assessed as his abilities decrease. Record the type of mobility equipment used. Is it a walking aid, wheelchair or powered wheelchair? Check whether any alterations or additions are needed for the equipment to improve mobility or posture.

Another area of mobility that needs to be assessed is the type of transport that the person uses to get to other locations. This needs to be examined to ensure that the person is travelling safely and is using safe equipment and safe methods of transport.

## POSTURE

Due to the progressive nature of this condition, close monitoring of the individual's posture is essential in order to minimise the effect of the muscle weakness. Good body alignment is important for maintaining the vital chest capacity for breathing. Note any asymmetry, contractures or deformity present.

## HOME SEATING

Initially, a child may not have any special seating but note their posture while seated, as this may indicate that they may need seating for postural support. If they have special seating, whether it is a home chair or a wheelchair, check that it is still providing the postural support required and that there is pressure relief in the chair if it is needed.

## UPPER-LIMB FUNCTION

Movement in the upper limbs is preserved for longer than in other areas of the body. As weakness increases and movement is reduced, the young person will use many compensatory strategies to preserve function. It is important to minimise loss of function as a consequence of contractures for as long as possible. Observation of the young person performing various tasks will reveal a great deal of information. Range of movement from shoulder to finger and range of movement in the hand should both be assessed.

## PERSONAL CARE

Each individual will need different levels of support to complete personal-care tasks. Therefore, each task has to be looked at individually to find out how long it takes to perform, as this will give an indication of the level of assistance that may be needed from parents and carers. It will also reveal how much effort the individual has to expend to complete the task.

## EATING AND DRINKING SKILLS

There are many aspects of eating and drinking that have to be assessed. Does the person have the hand and arm range of movement to get the food and the drink to their mouth? Do they have the strength to cut up their food and to lift their cup or cutlery to their mouth? Do they need special equipment to eat independently, such as mobile arm supports or elevated eating surfaces? Do they have to be fed? Do they have problems chewing and swallowing? Note should also be taken of any appetite changes, their normal diet and the consistency of the food they need. Another issue relating to eating is the weight of the person, as being overweight for people with Duchenne muscular dystrophy can cause extra problems.

## DRESSING

When looking at the individual's functional ability to dress, it is appropriate to observe the abilities of a younger child trying to dress. With the older child, it is more appropriate check the level of assistance that the individual requires as well as the degree of moving and handling necessary to get dressed and undressed. Some consideration should be given to the type of clothes selected in relation to comfort and ease of dressing. Clothes should be age-appropriate and should reflect the image that the individual wishes to convey.

## BATHING

When assessing bathing, consideration has to be given to the environment in which the person with muscular dystrophy bathes and whether there are any risks to the person while they are bathing. Consideration also has to be given to who assists them to bathe. It is important to know whether they use a shower or a bath, as the different methods of washing bring different problems. Trying to step into a bath is a big problem for a child with Duchenne muscular dystrophy but trying to maintain balance on a wet slippery floor is equally difficult and can be dangerous. In the later stages of the illness, it is necessary to document the type of equipment that is used and who is using the equipment.

## TOILETING

The issues with toileting include recording any bladder or bowel problems, as this can influence therapy. Detail any special equipment used and note whether anyone assists to toilet. Is the toilet a normal toilet or a wash–dry toilet? Do they always use the toilet or do they use a bottle or a sheath? Do they need postural support to sit over the toilet and do they have any pressure issues while sitting on the toilet?

## SELF-CARE

Other areas that have to be looked at regarding personal care are things like brushing teeth and grooming hair. Shaving can also be a problem for these young men. Note whether they use any special equipment to carry out these tasks or whether a carer performs them for the individual.

## SLEEP

Record the quality of sleep that the person gets and how many times a night the person's and carer's sleep is disturbed. If possible, try to establish what is causing the sleep disturbances. Is it respiratory, dietary, pain-related or psychological? Check whether the bed used is a standard or specialist bed. Does it meet the needs of the individual and their carers? It is also necessary to check whether the mattress has pressure-relieving qualities or whether they are using a sleep system to provide positioning support.

## SEXUALITY

With young adults, this needs to be addressed. It is not just about the sexual act. It may be about how medication or incontinence issues affect this aspect of their life. It is also about how they view themselves as a sexual person. Do they think they are attractive, etc.? Their parents' attitudes also have to be assessed, as they may not be aware that the young man wishes to express his sexuality.

## MOVING AND HANDLING

The amount of moving and handling that has to be undertaken to perform personal-care tasks also has to be assessed and note should be taken of any moving and handling equipment that is used in each task.

## DOMESTIC CHORES

Establish what chores the person with muscular dystrophy wants to participate in and find out who is responsible for carrying out the domestic chores. Who does the banking and shopping?

## SCHOOL AND NURSERY ASSESSMENTS

Personal-care issues will also have to be looked at in school and nursery, as will the areas in which personal care is carried out. Establish what support is available for the child in school and who provides assistance especially for personal-care issues.

## BUILDING

The school building needs to be checked to discover which areas of the school are accessible to the individual and to ascertain whether any building adaptations are required.

## CLASSROOMS

All subject classrooms need to be inspected to make sure that there is good access into the classroom and that the desks and equipment required can be reached by the individual with muscular dystrophy.

## FINE-MOTOR ACTIVITIES

The ability to carry out fine-motor school activities like handwriting and keyboard skills needs to be monitored. Care should be taken so that the child is positioned properly to carry out fine-motor tasks.

## SCHOOL SUBJECTS

Check what adjustments have been made to subject classes to allow the child to participate.

## COGNITION AND VISUAL PERCEPTUAL PROBLEMS

Does the child have the ability to remember instructions, concentrate on tasks and make safe judgements? Do they have any problems with the visual interpretation of what they are seeing or with spatial relationships?

## PEER GROUP

Is the child given the opportunity to mix with their peers at break times and does their peer group accept them?

## ACCESS TO SCHOOL OUTINGS

Are there provisions in place to allow them to participate in school outings?

## RECREATION

Find out what hobbies and leisure pursuits interest the person and what obstacles may prevent them from participating in leisure activities. How do they spend their free time? Do they have any pets?

## WORK

Find out what the individual's expectations are regarding paid or voluntary employment. If they are in employment, do any modifications need to be made to their workplace or their working practices?

## OTHER PROFESSIONALS AND AGENCIES

It is important to note any other professionals or agencies that are currently involved with the young person, such as consultants, therapists and social work colleagues. Good multidisciplinary working cannot be over-emphasised with this client group, as their problems are often multiple and interrelated. The therapist must know when to refer on to colleagues and other service providers. Below is a list of those who may have involvement with the young person. This is by no means exhaustive:

- general practitioner;
- health visitor;
- educational psychologist;
- pre-school visiting teacher;

- orthopaedic surgeon;
- neurologist;
- geneticist;
- dietician;
- speech therapist;
- community occupational therapist;
- social worker;
- family-care officer – Muscular Dystrophy Campaign;
- respite;
- community-care agencies;
- befriender services;
- housing services;
- hospice;
- physiotherapist;
- education services;
- architects, builders and similar agencies.

## FREQUENCY OF ASSESSMENT

An occupational therapy assessment or review of the young person should be carried out at least annually. More frequent reviews may be necessary at times of change, such as following periods of ill health or after surgery and following loss of ambulation.

## PLANNING

Following the assessment process, short and long-term occupational therapy goals have to be set with the individual and the family. These goals must be based on the person's preferences. Once goals are established, the occupational therapist will have to decide which occupational therapy service can best meet these goals. If an occupational therapist from a social work service has carried out an assessment at home and recognised that most of the issues identified by the family concern school or wheelchair issues, it may be more appropriate to ask an occupational therapist working in these fields to address these issues. Each therapist then needs to work out what interventions will meet the goals of the family.

## INTERVENTIONS

Interventions are the activities and actions that can assist the family to meet their goals. The following is an overview of some of the occupational therapy interventions that can assist people affected by Duchenne muscular dystrophy.

Some of these interventions will be discussed in greater detail in subsequent chapters.

## POSTURAL MANAGEMENT

Boys with Duchenne muscular dystrophy can develop spinal problems fairly quickly once they stop walking, so they need good postural management interventions to slow down the rate of spinal curvature (Turner et al., 2002). Postural management is an approach to the handling, treatment and positioning of children and adults with muscular dystrophy that will reduce the risk of contractures and the development of postural deformities. Passive and active movements of limbs will also slow down the development of contractures.

Good positioning will allow the person to carry out everyday activities with more ease and without adopting abnormal postures. If postural problems are not addressed, it can lead to pain, spinal problems and breathing difficulties.

The main pieces of equipment that can help with postural management are:

• sleep systems;
• postural seating;
• wheelchairs with postural seating systems;
• splints/orthotics.

## PAIN AND FATIGUE MANAGEMENT

There are a number of interventions that occupational therapists can suggest that can help with pain management. This may be the provision of pressure-relief equipment, such as the following:

• mattress;
• seating and wheelchair seating;
• pressure cushions for commodes, shower chairs and baths;
• padded and sheepskin slings.

Energy-conservation methods can be used, according to Birkholtz et al. (2004), to reduce pain by planning and pacing activities. Some methods of saving energy are listed below:

• If it is not important to the individual to do the task, can someone else do the work?
• Does the task need to be done every day?
• Spread the tasks over the whole day rather than trying to do everything in one time period.
• Can any tools, equipment or adaptations make the tasks easier?

Stress reduction and relaxation techniques can also help with pain management.

## HOUSING, SCHOOL AND WORKPLACE ADAPTATIONS

There are many housing adaptations that the therapist can recommend, according to Clutton et al. (2006). They can also help to obtain funding for adaptations that will make life easier for the person with muscular dystrophy and their carers. A few are listed below:

- ramps;
- bathroom alterations;
- extensions;
- handrails;
- door alterations;
- tracking hoists;
- lifts.

## EQUIPMENT

Occupational therapists can advise and provide many pieces of equipment (Pain et al., 2003) that can help the person to maintain their independence in daily living tasks, school tasks or work tasks. Equipment can also help the carer with their care tasks. The following are a minute selection of the equipment that could assist a person with muscular dystrophy:

- hoists and slings;
- shower chairs;
- bath lifts;
- eating aids;
- toilet equipment;
- writing aids.

## MOVING AND HANDLING INFORMATION AND EQUIPMENT

Information and training on how to move and handle an individual can be offered by the occupational therapists, along with advice on equipment that can help when transferring the individual from one position to another (College of Occupational Therapists, 2006b). Some of the common moving and handling equipment supplied by therapists are listed below:

- transfer boards;
- hoists and slings;
- sliding sheets;
- handling belts.

## WHEELCHAIR PROVISION

Most wheelchair-provision services employ occupational therapists who are involved in the assessment and provision of wheelchairs. They may also have to train the individual in how to use their wheelchair. The therapist will have to give recommendations regarding the postural support and pressure relief required for the chair, as well as the type of controls needed to operate the wheelchair. Other occupational therapists may have to provide similar information to allow the individuals to purchase a wheelchair or to obtain charity funding for a chair.

## TRANSPORT ISSUES

The therapist, as well as providing particulars about suitable car seats, harnesses and vehicles, can supply advice on safe ways to transport individuals. They can also suggest car modifications. Occupational therapists can also give out information on mobility benefits, parking badges and parking bays (Turner et al., 2002).

## TEACHING NEW METHODS

Everyone is used to carrying out activities in their own way. An occupational therapist can look at how the individual carries out a task and suggest alternative ways to do it. This may allow the person to complete the task independently. Examples are:

- teaching a person to get dressed on the bed if they have balance problems;
- using a computer to do homework as opposed to having to write it all by hand;
- substitute a battery-operated toothbrush for an ordinary toothbrush.

## SUPPORT GROUPS

Many occupational therapists can provide information about and links to support groups for the individuals with Duchenne muscular dystrophy, their parents or their siblings.

## ENVIRONMENTAL CONTROL SYSTEMS

Systems that let the individual with muscular dystrophy control their own home environment can be accessed via the occupational therapist. These systems can control heating, lighting, opening doors and electrical appliances like televisions and computers (Harmer & Bakheit, 1999).

## SKIN PROTECTION AND MANAGEMENT

It is vital to ensure that any equipment issued will not damage the individual's skin. This can happen if the individual is allergic to synthetics or any of the materials that are used to make the equipment. If the skin is vulnerable, pressure-relieving materials should be used (Harpin, 2003) where the skin comes into contact with the equipment and measures should be taken to limit moving and handling tasks. The number of moving and handling activities a person with Duchenne muscular dystrophy may have to tolerate every day may be a factor that can cause skin problems. It is advisable to review how the person is moved and how many times a day he has to be moved, as it may be possible to change the methods of handling to reduce skin contact or to reduce the number of times the person is handled throughout the day.

If the individual wears splints, ensure that these are not causing marking or chaffing of the skin. Providing advice on suitable but appropriate clothes and shoes for the individual can also reduce skin problems. Another area to watch for is skin breakdown on young men who wear masks on their face during ventilation. These can often cause skin problems. Advice on changing the individual's position when seated in one chair or a bed for long periods of time will also help to prevent skin problems. This can be made easier for the carer and the individual by providing adjustable beds and tilt-in-space chairs so that the area that pressure is on can be changed easily with the push of a button.

## ACCESS TO PLAY EQUIPMENT

It is important that boys with Duchenne muscular dystrophy have the opportunity to play to develop their skills. Occupational therapists can suggest toys and activities that will help with their development (Parham & Fazio, 1997).

## IT EQUIPMENT: HARDWARE AND SOFTWARE

If an individual cannot use a standard mouse and keyboard, details of alternative types of keyboards, word-recognition software and joysticks can be supplied. If they are having problems with software programs, alternative types of program can be sought.

## ACCESSING THE EDUCATIONAL CURRICULUM

The occupational therapists can advise teachers on alternative ways for the boy with muscular dystrophy to be able to participate in school work. This could be asking for handouts to be provided or for scribers to assist when the boy is having problems writing or it could be providing book supports, etc. Equally, it could be the provision of suitable-height desks and chairs with postural support (Muscular Dystrophy Campaign, 2004b).

## COMMUNITY-CARE SERVICES

Planning and organising funding for community-care services is a fundamental element of occupational therapy interventions. These can be home-care services, respite care and major adaptations (Dimond, 2004).

## CARING FOR THE CAREGIVERS

Occupational therapists also have a duty of care to ensure the needs of the parents and carers are addressed separately from those of the person with Duchenne muscular dystrophy.

## BENEFITS ADVICE AND REPORTS

Information about the benefits that the individual and the family could be entitled to should always be provided. The occupational therapist may also have to support benefit claims for the family by providing detailed reports on the individual and their needs.

The above interventions are some of the many ways that occupational therapists can be of assistance to people with Duchenne muscular dystrophy and their families.

## EVALUATION

Once the actions and programmes have been put in place, the occupational therapist needs to make sure that these interventions are fulfilling the original goals set by the individual and their carers following the assessment process. If their goals have not been met, the therapist will have to re-evaluate their treatment plan and seek alternative ways for the person with muscular dystrophy to achieve their goals.

## KEY POINTS

- Occupational therapists have a unique role in supporting and working with young men with Duchenne muscular dystrophy and their families.
- Occupational therapists can be employed by a number of different agencies, with each agency being responsible for providing separate services.
- Occupational therapy is a health profession concerned with promoting health and well-being through occupation.
- Occupation is central to normal human existence and its absence is a threat to health.
- Occupational therapy is a process of assessment, planning, intervention and evaluation.
- The main goal of assessment in occupational therapy is to get a clear understanding of the individual, their social circumstances and their environment in order to develop a treatment plan.

- Good multidisciplinary working cannot be over-emphasised with this client group.
- Treatment goals must be based on the person's preferences.
- Interventions are the activities and actions that can assist the family to meet their goals.
- All treatment programmes have to be evaluated.

## CASE STUDY

### REFERRAL

The local mainstream primary school contacted the social services occupational therapist for advice regarding taking a boy with Duchenne muscular dystrophy on a proposed school outing to the cinema and ice rink.

### ASSESSMENTS REQUIRED

- child's attitude to the proposed trip;
- school staff's attitude to taking the child on the trip;
- environmental assessment of the leisure complex building which housed the cinema and the ice rink, including auditorium, toilet areas, foyer and parking facilities;
- suitable parking near the complex;
- the chair the child would use on the ice rink;
- the best time of day to arrange the outing if there are fatigue issues.

### PLAN AND INTERVENTIONS

The goal was for the child to attend the outing with the rest of the class. To be able to achieve this one goal, the following intervention issues would have to be addressed by the therapist:

- bus with tail lift was provided and funded by the education department, with a driver who was trained in how to position the boy and his wheelchair safely in the vehicle;
- special-needs auxiliary accompanied the boy on the bus and was willing to assist with personal care, including feeding, on the outing;
- small portable hoist and sling provided by social services to take on the outing to allow the child to transfer into the chair used on the ice and the toilet, if this was necessary;
- transportation of any personal-care or medical equipment that may be needed during the outing;
- the best time of day to arrange the outing if there are fatigue issues.

EVALUATION

The child enjoyed the outing, but felt that he missed out, as he did not get to travel on the coach with the rest of his friends. On future outings, arrangements will be made for some of the child's friends to travel in the tail-lift bus with him.


## STUDY QUESTIONS

- What considerations should you take into account when using standardised tests?
- What is the philosophy of occupational therapy?
- Where do occupational therapists work?
- Why is it necessary to carry out assessments?
- What interventions can help with pain management?

# 3 The Psychosocial and Emotional Impact of Duchenne Muscular Dystrophy: Some Considerations

CLAIRE TESTER

## INTRODUCTION

The diagnosis of Duchenne muscular dystrophy can occur at different times: at birth, if there is a significant family history; or later, at the preschool stage, when motor milestones appear delayed; or when the boy falls, about five years of age, seemingly clumsy and stands up by 'walking up' his legs (called Gower's manoeuvre). At diagnosis, the prognosis is usually made, too. Until recently, the prognosis was given until the mid or late teen years. However, with the introduction of Bi-Pap and C-Pap (continuous airway pressure) as overnight ventilation, the prognosis has been extended into the twenties and thirties. It is still being challenged, with men living into their forties in Scandinavia (Eagle, 2002).

Such men are living independently, working, some married and some fathers. The overnight ventilation has been introduced over recent years and is not yet standard practice. However, many parents still understand their son's prognosis to be in the teens and this belief shadows their lives. When working with a boy who has Duchenne muscular dystrophy and with his family, it is necessary to consider the emotional and psychosocial impact of the condition. It is easier to address only the physical and environmental needs, which are practical and more easily assessed, but this is only part of the therapy that you can provide. An occupational therapist is trained to look holistically at an individual and this is especially so when working with children and their families.

The emotional and psychological impact of a life-limiting condition should not be underestimated (Tester, 2006). As it is a deteriorating condition, there are constant changes, which can be viewed as a series of losses, of ability and skills. With the introduction of overnight ventilation and the possibility of longer lives, it is necessary to encourage thinking for planning for the future, as most families would, such as higher education, independent living and having meaningful adult relationships. Such thinking needs to be encouraged at an early stage, namely at primary school, for the benefit of the child and family. The expectation of the son dying in his teens has resulted in an unintentional waiting. As one mother described:

'It feels as if my life has been "on hold" because I'd made up my mind to do anything for my son in the time he has up until his 20's and then I would do things for me. I get up at 5.30am to get him dressed, washed and toileted for the school bus, and sleep near him in the night for when he needs turning. My husband didn't understand and didn't like it so we split up. There are a lot of things I want to do but I will have time when my son is not here.'

How parents react, their expectations and their coping strategies directly affect their son (Sterken, 1996). The emotional guilt felt by parents to care for their son may result in what may be regarded as over-protective behaviour. It is not unusual to encounter boys who present as emotionally immature. Conversely, some boys may present as more mature than their years for different reasons, such as being in predominantly adult company, and having knowledge of their condition. Frustration and anger can boil over:

'He rams his power chair into the walls when he is angry. He has real outbursts and takes chunks out of the walls with his footplates. Sometimes he'll run at his brother in an argument. He can be very aggressive with that chair.'
(Mother of 12-year-old boy with Duchenne muscular dystrophy).

First and foremost, a boy with Duchenne muscular dystrophy is a growing boy, with the usual emotions and developing hormones but who will become more physically dependent as he grows. This physical dependency and the awareness of his condition will affect his emotional and psychological well-being. It is important to see the person first and the condition second. How one works as a therapist and is accepted by the boy and his family depend upon your approach and sensitivity. Some points to consider follow. They are not applicable to every family but are to help when thinking about what might be happening to the lad and his family. This may explain why a piece of equipment or planning a home extension, etc. can prove difficult to consider and accept for parents, and their son. It is necessary to look at the wider context, to ask about concerns and, if need be, the fears when blocks are encountered. An attitude by the therapist of ambivalence, such as 'Well, if you don't want it, there's nothing I can do for you', or of dogma, such as 'He needs the chair now and will have to have that one', will only alienate the family and boy. Such attitudes are not necessary and are only borne out of ignorance by the therapist. Families need preparation and supported guidance as to what each age and stage will bring (Bluebond-Langner, 2000). Thinking and consideration on the part of the therapist can contribute to a more meaningful and effective therapeutic approach.

## SOME CONSIDERATIONS AT DIFFERENT AGES AND STAGES

The age of a child with Duchenne muscular dystrophy is linked to a different stage in development (motor and emotional) and of the condition. Here is an overview of considerations which may be factors at each age and stage.

### INFANT

Diagnosis at the infant stage affects the parent and their relationship with their baby. It is the loss of the 'normal' expected baby which is experienced and an adjustment to the thought of a future disability. Parents may experience anxiety or ambivalence towards their baby as they come to terms with the diagnosis. Babies are sensitive to their mother's emotions particularly and may present with difficulties in feeding, sleeping or behaviour (Winnicott, 1967). The infant does not present with specific condition-related difficulties at this stage, although there may be a referral to an occupational therapist and/or physiotherapist for support in motor milestones after the first year. It should be recognised that it is the parent who particularly needs the support.

### PRE-SCHOOL

The child is active and mobile, with some delay in motor milestones. Developmentally, they are exploring the world around them. Diagnosis at this stage does not lessen the shock for the parents, as one mother said when her two toddler sons were diagnosed: 'I lost my little boys on that day and the men they would become.'

Information for nursery staff with parents' consent may be helpful, as the boy may be perceived as being deliberately slow in physical activities, but the full diagnosis and prognosis do not need to be shared with the staff.

### PRIMARY SCHOOL

It is during this stage that changes are most dramatic. This comes at a time at which the child is entering a new environment and making friends. Frequent falling occurs at about five years, and a manual self-propelling wheelchair is usually introduced at around eight or nine years. This affects environmental access at home and school, and social activities. Frustration and a real sense of loss may be experienced by the child. Some children present as withdrawn. Taunting and some bullying of the boy may occur. Carers are introduced for toileting needs at school. This is the start of the boy's body becoming unpredictable, as muscle power is lost. Losing skills affects the boy's confidence and self-esteem. His body image is affected.

## SECONDARY SCHOOL

Entering school, the young boy appears physically different in his wheelchair amongst his peers. He becomes more dependent for basic self-care needs, such as toileting and self-feeding. The independence of the adolescent is removed over time as he becomes more dependent upon friends and carers to collect lunch, cut it up, help with feeding, getting books from class, holding open doors, etc. The environmental limitations further compound the sense of difference – peers running up stairs whilst the teenager with Duchenne muscular dystrophy waits for the lift, or waits at the bottom of the stairs without access, for example.

School outings can be planned without consideration, e.g. for coach access, and the teenager can be left out. The young adult becomes increasingly dependent, losing his upper-limb abilities, as his peers become more independent, with increased responsibilities.

Appearance becomes more important in the teenage years, as dressing like one's peers plays a significant part in group identity. Clothes chosen for ease of dressing and toileting can conflict with this. There is often embarrassment for the growing young man in being washed and dressed by female carers, and spontaneous penile erections can occur.

It is important to convey to a teenager a positive sense of what they can achieve, balanced with what they will be able to physically do. This can be difficult and there is a need for sensitivity by the therapist in supporting the parent in helping the teenage boy to make exam and career choices at 13 years. This will involve a sensitive discussion of projected loss of physical abilities in the late teens and early twenties. A neurological assessment of intellectual and cognitive abilities can be helpful (Cotton et al., 1998).


## HIGHER EDUCATION

It is important for the young adult to plan for the future and to consider options when at secondary school to look ahead. This is a positive aspect but requires sensitivity in realistic careers advice. Many young men pursue a career involving IT. Planning for a degree also requires consideration of the college's access and facilities available. As one young man commented, 'I got my place at college but as term began they said I couldn't attend all lectures because they were upstairs and there wasn't a lift. They knew I was coming, why didn't they consider that?' The degree of need for equipment, the degree of paralysis and consequent support for young men with Duchenne muscular dystrophy are not universally understood. The occupational therapist at school with the social services occupational therapist need to be involved as soon as possible when a course at college/university has been selected in order to plan equipment needs, access to the curriculum and physical access, including building of ramps, etc.

## LIVING INDEPENDENTLY

When a young man chooses to live independently, away from home, this can be seen as a rejection by his parents and a cause of real worry for them. There may be an emotional double bind for the man in wanting to live his own life, yet appreciating the love, care and time given to him by his parents. The parents may put up reasons for their son not being able to live independently, for rational as well as emotional reasons. Separation may be difficult and traumatic for both sides. For some families, the compromise of living next door to each other, or having a flat attached to the house, has been possible. The young man will need to be responsible for spending his disability benefit and for purchasing carer time, which involves interviewing and employing his own carers. (Housing requirements are discussed in Chapter 12.)

## OVERNIGHT VENTILATION

Overnight ventilation is introduced after sleep studies provide indicators. This is often in the mid to late teens. Sleep studies and ventilation may need to be explained to parents, even after the medical consultant has explained the process. For some parents, it is too much information to take in. For some young men, the introduction of Bi-Pap ventilation and the information that it will improve prognosis may be the first time that they become aware that they have a life-limiting condition. This results in understandable reactions of anger and shock on occasion, leading to a rejection of the ventilation equipment or an anxiety of depending on it, perceiving it as a life-saver.

## GRIEF AND LOSS

As the condition causes wasting from proximal muscle to distal muscles, motor skills and abilities are being lost as time progresses and the young man becomes paralysed with very limited movement, being able to move his head, fingers and toes. (If a spinal fusion has been performed, then there is restricted movement at the head.) Grief and loss are associated with bereavement but can be experienced about one's own life, in terms of present losses incurred, and the projected future life being lost. This is often perceived as being relevant to adults only, but children and young adults are able to experience such depth of feeling (Klein, 1988). 'I really miss walking,' said a 10-year-old boy with Duchenne muscular dystrophy, recently confined to a wheelchair. The loss of skills affects body image, too, and one's sense of self (Judd, 1995). In Duchenne muscular dystrophy, this series of losses can occur quickly over time and be difficult for the boy to come to terms with, as the ability to perform a task or hobby can be lost. One 12-year-old boy who was skilled in modelling clay lost the ability to mould with his hands, as he could neither support the clay nor make the required fine movements and although he persisted for a while, his attempts were clumsy and he quickly ceased.

Health professionals, as well as parents, may not comment on the ongoing loss of skills. One 12-year-old boy said, 'Look, I can't move my arms up to my head now. Why? No-one tells me why? Will I be able to do this again?' It is important to talk and listen to the boy, asking if anything has changed. This provides an opportunity for discussion. This may be continued with the parents, or the doctor, but dialogue needs to be started. Different parents choose what they wish their sons to know about their condition. Consequently, difficult questions can occur for the therapist, such as when friends with the same condition die. It is necessary to find out what is understood by the young man himself.

A therapist walking alongside a 16-year-old in his power chair said, 'We were going along the pavement when suddenly out of nowhere he said of a boy at his school, "He died. And he's got what I've got, D.M.D. Why did he die? Is that what's going to happen to me?"' In this instance, the therapist explained that everyone is different and put questions back to the boy to ask him what he knew about Duchenne muscular dystrophy and whom he felt he could ask about his own condition. The therapist suggested to the boy that she could speak to his parents and raise his need for more answers than she was able to provide. The young man was in agreement.

Pain can be experienced as total pain (Saunders, 1993), including emotional, physical, psychological and spiritual. A carer providing respite for a young man with Duchenne muscular dystrophy commented, 'It was already 11pm and it took myself and a colleague one and a half hours to get him just right and comfortable in bed. Just little movements which were hardly movements at all. He said he was in pain. Every time we said, "we'll say goodnight", he said it was something else that needed moving very slightly. You know, I think he didn't want to be left alone in the room. We left the door open and said we would pop in through the night even when he was asleep. That seemed to help. He needed comforting and reassurance but at 19 he couldn't ask for it I suppose.'

## DEPRESSION

Mood changes can occur in the normal course of childhood, adolescence and adulthood. However, a prolonged mood and associated behaviour such as loss of appetite can be an indicator of an anxiety or depression. Depression can be overlooked but should be taken seriously. The sense of isolation experienced by a young man with Duchenne muscular dystrophy can be reinforced as he loses muscle power and skills, and when friends or relatives with Duchenne muscular dystrophy die. There are also frustrations in daily life, and of being socially isolated by peers. Worries and concerns need to be recognised and discussed before depression becomes a real issue. There is often an assumption that someone else will identify a mental health problem, whether a member of the family, a health professional or a school counsellor. This is not always so. Occupational therapists are trained in both physical and psychiatric conditions, and respective therapeutic interventions, and can identify the need for screening and refer. References for guidelines and assessments are given at the end of this book.

## IMPACT ON PARENTS

The way in which the diagnosis and prognosis are given to the parent(s) affects the way in which a parent can feel supported (Sloper, 1996). As one mother described it, 'I felt abandoned and let loose with this frightening information about my beautiful baby. All I could do was cry. I felt very alone'. A doctor imparting the initial information may not be seen at the next hospital clinic, and a parent may wrongly believe that questions can only be answered by the hospital medical staff. This can contribute to parents feeling further unsupported. Parents can be encouraged to request a second follow-up appointment with the same doctor within a fortnight, or as a follow-up appointment by the general practitioner to discuss concerns further and to receive support. The diagnosis and prognosis can be experienced as shock and this includes denial, as well as anger with the doctor and health professionals. A father said, 'It was like they all knew about my son and I didn't. They knew what the condition was, and how it would go and I didn't. It was as if they were all colluding with each other. My boy was only 3 and was normal'. Parents use different defence and coping behaviours which are natural reactions that health professionals need to recognise, and not define parents as 'difficult', 'over reactive' or worse, but to exercise compassion and patience. Duchenne muscular dystrophy can act as a stressor upon the whole family and affect the dynamics of a family (Cadman et al., 1991). The working career of parents can be affected, as a parent may need to stay at home to provide care. Sometimes, a parent works part-time for suitability of hours rather than according to their own skills and abilities. Although this occurs for many parents whose children do not have Duchenne muscular dystrophy, it can be more fraught and continue far longer for parents of boys with Duchenne muscular dystrophy. This may have financial implications.

Parents are faced with practical day-to-day difficulties whilst trying to keep everything on an 'even keel'. The physical and emotional demands upon parents are considerable, and can lead to a depressive episode (Daoud et al., 2004). It can be difficult for a parent to consider their own health needs (MDA, 1998) and, at times, they can become overwhelmed. As one mother remarked, 'Every birthday becomes harder for me. I cannot hold back the time and I get so upset as each year means more deterioration. Yet he is so excited as his birthday comes up. Yes, I do the balloons and the cake, and the party, but I can see ahead, and I don't want to. I always get very tearful around his birthday and have to hide it'.

Parents need increasing support as their son becomes older to address social needs. Social isolation, depression and anger were identified as main concerns and difficulties by parents of sons with Duchenne muscular dystrophy by Bothwell et al. (2002).

## PSYCHOSOCIAL POINTERS TO CONSIDER

Some things to be aware of and keep in mind are:

• The importance of gaining trust with the parents and the boy/young man is fundamental to a good relationship and the foundation for therapeutic intervention. It is helpful not to cross the threshold for the first time with equipment. It can be retrieved from the car if essential. It will be necessary to establish what is understood of the condition by the family at regular intervals in order to support appropriately.

• Everyone is individual and unique and this includes coping behaviours and strategies. By talking to parents and the boy, together and separately, it is helpful to hear how they are coping (Katz, 2002).

• Independence and empowerment need to be encouraged. He has his own voice, which needs to be respected, and listened to.

• Being different – keep equipment to a minimum and as unobtrusive as possible.

• What is meaningful to the individual – it is not always the activities of daily living that the therapist identifies. Discuss with the boy what is important and relevant to him in a day, and in different environments.

• Choices – share information with the family of equipment on the market, as well as that which can be provided by the NHS/social services. As Philippa Harpin (Former OT Advisor to Muscular Dystrophy Campaign) once remarked, 'It's like cars; we all need to know what's on the market and decide whether to save up for the Porsche or whether the Skoda better suits our needs'.

• Looking different – clothes are important. Help with suggested designs on the market, such as tracksuit bottoms with poppers down the sides, as used by sportsmen.

• Recognise that there may be fear and anxiety related to loss of muscle power and skills. For example, one boy was trying to exercise as much as possible in the false belief that he could develop strength in his hands and upper limbs. This made him tired and exhausted, and is contra-indicated in Duchenne muscular dystrophy. Build trust and talk to the boy about his concerns and level of understanding. Always check with parents beforehand what they understand, and also what they wish their son to know of his condition. This can vary greatly.

- Difficulties in making and keeping friends. 'I don't go out so much now because my friends like to climb trees and I have to wait at the bottom and they drop things on me,' said one 10-year-old.
- Anger and frustration. How does the boy, and young adult, express anger? One teacher reported, 'He has to stay in as he runs his chair into the other children in the playground'. She did not recognise his frustration nor the provocation of the boy by his peers. It is necessary to look past the surface. Anger can be channelled in a healthy way and involve others in sport and play. This may involve help with social skills.
- Expressing feelings and concerns. The young man can be caught in an emotional double bind of not wishing to upset his parents and will mask his own feelings of despondency or sadness by smiling and presenting as easy to please. Who can listen? This might be a carer at school. However, such a close relationship is not continued from primary to secondary school. It is helpful to speak to the carer(s) who are often in need of support themselves and unsure of what to do with a boy's concerns.
- Aspect of the boy/young man perceiving himself as the cause of a secondary trauma to the family, sensing himself as a burden, making the lives of his parents and siblings difficult, such as the family transport being a van, of equipment in the home, or having to move to adapted housing (Mannoni, 1987).
- The fear of dying underlies anxiety. Such anxiety may be seen as panic, e.g. as when there is a chest infection. It is helpful to discuss this separately with the young man, and his parents.
- There may be a depression when the boy or teenager presents with a flat affect. This needs to be addressed. There may be a sense of pointlessness, of powerlessness and of not perceiving anything positive in life. Depression is real and should not be disregarded. (See references for depression and anxiety at the end of this book.)
- Limiting appetite. A possible anorexia or self-starvation can occur, partly because it becomes more difficult to eat a meal and takes a long time. Meals can become cold, and friends can move off to something else at school, resulting in the young adult picking at his food and not eating very much. Often, meals are not fully eaten. Some young men are aware of their weight when a parent insists on physically lifting them. Consequently, the young man tries to limit his weight by not eating very much in order to be lighter. For some young men, their Duchenne muscular dystrophy causes them to become overweight and they are often accused of being fat and overeating, which is not the case. It is also necessary to consider that some boys and young adults do not eat at school, as they wish to avoid being toileted at school during the day and all the embarrassment that this incurs is avoided

by them. This is worth investigating, as attitudes of teachers or lack of appropriate provision can be discovered. One boy of 14 said, 'I wait till I get home now. I can't put my hand up anymore and I have to ask. It's really embarrassing and my teacher usually tells me to wait when I can't'. This aspect of toileting is not always asked and yet is a common problem. A parent commented of her 12-year-old son, 'He's bursting when he gets home and he has to go straight to the toilet. He has soiled himself in the past and I know he's so embarrassed by this. I don't think he eats at school either because he is so hungry and thirsty when he gets home. I don't know how he can think and do his work properly without proper food and drink'.

- Potential conflict can occur when a parent, often the mother, has a difficulty in acknowledging her son as an independent young man. Some parents use baby monitors, or sleep near their sons. It is as if there is a secondary weaning (Lanyado & Horne, 1999) which needs to occur, as a parent finds separation difficult. This is reinforced by the young man being physically dependent for all of his needs, imitating an earlier stage of development. It is important not to judge but to help parents and their son find age-appropriate ways.

- How is the boy/young man with Duchenne muscular dystrophy viewed by his siblings? Siblings can react in different ways and at different times. It may be pity, over-protection, resentment or ambivalence. One mother explained, 'I got there just in time as his brother was operating the hoist for him and they were arguing so much that his brother was threatening to leave him up in the air and wouldn't help him!'

- School teachers. It is key to actively involve teachers in planning independence at school. Sometimes, there is a misunderstanding of the condition of Duchenne muscular dystrophy by the staff. The condition is seen but not the person behind it. Having a child/young adult with a disability in the class can provoke a lot of anxiety for teaching staff.

- A child/young adult, and his parents, can become overwhelmed by all of the specialist input: occupational therapist, physiotherapist, social services occupational therapist, the muscular dystrophy family officer, dietician, carers, hospital visits to clinic and consultant doctor. It is helpful to establish how many visitors there are to the house and to coordinate these as a wider team, and to identify overlap and sharing of information. Conversely, it can work the other way when a young man leaves school and therapy services are not as frequent or are negligible.

- Family holidays can become fraught or not take place at all. Advice and information on holidays and breaks with disabled facilities should be given freely rather than requested. This enables the family to plan ahead, and to be aware of different facilities.

- There is often an increasing lack of spontaneity for the young man with Duchenne muscular dystrophy and this is to be discouraged, as it is part of youth. The young man may be dependent upon his family for an activity.

Local voluntary agencies and services may be helpful. Again information on activities and access needs to be given freely rather than waiting for a difficulty or frustration to arise.

- As the young man reaches his late teens, his paralysis affects all four limbs and leaves only the inter and distal phalangeal joints in his hands and the distal joints in his metatarsals in his feet with the ability to move independently. It is important to remember that his mind is active.

## EMOTIONAL IMPACT UPON THERAPIST

To work with a child or adolescent who has a life-limiting condition, which is also a deteriorating one, impacts on the therapist, whichever therapy field they work in, be it community, school, social services, hospital or hospice. Some therapists find it very difficult at the outset and it is realistic to acknowledge if they cannot work with the child and family. This decision should be respected. It should be acknowledged that the therapist working with the child/young adult needs support from colleagues.

Some thoughts for the therapist are:

- It is necessary to show compassion and sensitivity rather than sympathy and pity. These last two are not helpful and singularly patronising.
- Do not over-identify with the boy and his family. Recognise and reflect upon your own feelings. Consciously raising one's own feelings in private, although painful, is helpful, as one's own feelings can unconsciously and actively interfere with one's therapeutic approach (Bye, 1998).
- It can be difficult for the therapist to plan and set therapy goals when the boy/young adult is losing skills. This can result in the therapist feeling de-skilled. It is necessary to plan with the boy/young adult on what is meaningful and to structure any therapy around maintaining independence in a deteriorating condition. This can be challenging when in parallel with the active growing and developing of the boy into a young adult.
- Do not be hard on yourself. There will be days which are difficult and the sense of frustration may feel overwhelming. In this way, it can echo that of the young man and can be helpful in gaining insight. No one therapist has all of the answers and can put everything right, as life is not like that.
- Some therapists may experience, although not witness, the young man dying. This is not something to be feared or ignored. It may be helpful to attend the funeral, to send a card to the parents or to visit them. It is important to acknowledge the young man both for oneself and for the family. Without some sort of resolution, it may detrimentally affect how the therapist works with another boy or young man with Duchenne muscular dystrophy. We are all human but occasionally can try to be 'professional', which can be misinterpreted as denying one's feelings.

## KEY POINTS

• It is necessary to consider the emotional and psychosocial impact of the condition.
• How parents react, their expectations and coping strategies directly affect their son in terms of his own coping behaviour and future plans. Parents need support, too.
• A boy with Duchenne muscular dystrophy is a growing boy, with normal emotions and developing hormones, but who will become more physically dependent as he grows. This dependency will affect him emotionally and psychologically.
• Families need support at each stage and age. Thinking and consideration by the therapist can contribute to a more meaningful and effective therapeutic approach.
• Grief and loss can be experienced about one's own life, in terms of skills lost and a projected lost future. Any prolonged mood changes and associated behaviour can be indicators of anxiety, or depression, and need to be recognised.
• The therapist can be affected emotionally, too.

## CASE STUDY

Two parents have two small boys, and the youngest son is diagnosed with Duchenne muscular dystrophy at two years of age when his motor milestones are delayed. He is assessed by the paediatric occupational therapist. This therapist is part of a review in imparting the diagnosis to the mother, which is given by the paediatrician. With parental consent, the other son is referred for genetic testing, but does not have Duchenne muscular dystrophy.

The occupational therapist is involved with programme planning at home and at the nursery. She provides guidance on helping the child and acknowledging some gross motor problems, but does not impart the diagnosis to nursery staff, in accordance with the mother's wishes. Both parents are naturally full of questions and distressed.

After discussion with the head occupational therapist, the therapist seeks supervision from a psychologist for her discussions with the mother, who is having real difficulties in coming to terms with the diagnosis, presenting as emotionally distraught.

With the parents, the occupational therapist discusses their need for answers to questions that she is unable to answer. With their consent, she raises this with the general practitioner and the paediatrician, who invite the parents to contact and arrange an appointment to discuss their concerns with one of them. The occupational therapist also explores the possibility of the parents contacting a counsellor at the medical practice to discuss their emotions in more depth than the occupational therapist can offer. The trust and relationship that the occupational therapist has built up over a few weeks enable the mother to recognise this need. The father is not ready to meet a counsellor, he says.

The occupational therapist withdraws, as early therapy intervention with the child has been achieved. The parents and nursery staff have a contact telephone number for the occupational therapist if there are any specific difficulties arising.

## STUDY QUESTIONS

• Consider whether it is necessary to give the diagnosis to nursery staff, and why the mother felt this would have a negative effect upon her son.
• What is understood by 'seeking supervision'? What guidance could be expected from the psychologist to the occupational therapist and how would this be helpful?
• Consider the approach used by the occupational therapist here and how this might affect the future relationship with occupational therapy as the young boy deteriorates.
• Explore coping and defence behaviours which might be used by the parents, and the therapist.

# 4 From Our Point of View: From Young Men with Duchenne Muscular Dystrophy, as Shared with Claire

## CLAIRE TESTER

The following first piece was written by Daniel Morrison for this book.

I was born in 1985, perfectly healthy. My infant years went by rather insignificantly, although to my mother the sight of my first step and the sound of my first word would turn out to be far from insignificant considering what was around the corner.

My nursery leaders noticed something slightly different in my movement from the other children's. Being the age I was meant that I was unaware of what exactly was happening, so things progressed and a year or so later a diagnosis arrived – Duchenne Muscular Dystrophy.

I was in primary one of my education, so like any other child that just wanted to go and play I took it in my stride. Then again it didn't really matter because I doubt it would have made sense to me anyway.

The further I got into primary, the more I understood what was happening with me. However whilst I clearly had slight physical difficulties, I was treated without any prejudice, after all children don't really have life experience to judge one of their own – adults on the other hand treated me slightly differently, but to this day I can't put my finger on exactly what it was.

I often got frustrated with myself. Football, as with many boys, was my first love. I was slowly losing my ability to run and I began to fall over quite often. When out playing football at school, I was helped back up on to my feet by my classmates. I was assigned a teaching auxiliary to aid me around school. At that point I felt like people were starting to show concern, concern that I felt was rather unjust.

Gradually I became accustomed to having my auxiliary around. Having her around ended up being something required by me. 1996, my second week back at school after the Christmas and New Year holiday was to be a monumental week and year in my life; the most traumatic year of my life and my last week of school that I could walk unaided.

Whilst visiting family friends I had fallen and broken my leg. A rather innocuous fall that on any other day wouldn't have even registered as a serious fall landed me in hospital. I was very aware that this could be my last action on my feet. Many tears resulted from my leg break, less for the pain than you would believe. A week on and I was back at school. Two or so months and four leg casts later, the uncertain and arduous task of me getting back upon my feet began to gain speed.

I was introduced to two pieces of equipment that if I never ever saw again would be too soon, even though I understand they were of major importance in getting me back on my feet. The full length leg splints and the standing frame. My final primary year had rolled around, at this stage the leg splints were working a treat and I was managing to stand and take steps. But every time I took some confidence, something would come along and take the shine off it. Was it losing my balance whilst trying to stand independently? Was it getting a new shiny wheelchair delivered while still trying my hardest to get on my feet – making me question whether or not people had confidence in me ever walking again? Eventually November 1996 arrived and a strong realisation that my fight to gain my ability to walk independently wasn't really going anywhere. I had lost my fight, valiantly.

First year of high school, is generally a difficult time for anyone. Here is where the ill-fated standing frame made its entrance. The leg splints were becoming less favourable also. Physiotherapy was obviously an integral addition to my routine; my knees were in a constantly bent position due to my seating position. The splints were designed to straighten the knees – however they had begun to resist the pressure thus putting me in great pain. So envisage if you would, my legs straightened to their limits, two people lifting me by my shoulders to an upright standing position on legs in extreme pain already, then from this into a frame with Velcro straps around my thighs and back. The frame was on wheels; I was unbelievably rolled into classroom – up the front – and was expected to work through the excruciating pain I was in. I was taken out of the classroom and put back in my chair, after which I would look at the exhausted people who had put me back in my chair and see that they couldn't stand doing that again – not due to their exhaustion but due to seeing me in pain.

Thankfully, for all concerned neither piece of equipment was ever used again.


## AGED 11 YEARS

'I don't like school, it's difficult. My teacher is nice though. I am in a small class (for learning difficulties). I don't like maths, and I don't like writing. My teacher says my handwriting is messy, so I try very hard, but my hand does get tired. I used to exercise my arms, you know like a muscle man, to make them stronger but my physio said not to. My arms aren't very strong really. It takes me a while to push myself in my chair. Sometimes someone else pushes me but in the playground I can't keep up with the others. That makes me fed up.

I've got some friends at school, in my class. And at home I play outside. It's usually football, but Jamie (friend) gets cross because the football gets stuck under my footplates. Mum says she's going to get a big football that won't get stuck. That would be good. Mum doesn't want me to go out when it is raining, or when it's really cold. Jamie comes over to my house and we play on the computer. I've got a cool game he hasn't got. No, I don't really go to his house because it's got two big steps at the front door, and steps at the back. Mum can't carry me on her own, and Jamie's Mum says she's worried she'll drop me. So I have to wait for Jamie's Dad to get home. When Jamie had a party last year though his Dad carried me into the house, and I sat on the sofa. With cushions. His Mum said I could do the music for the games. I got them out in the Bumps (Musical Bumps) really quickly!

At home Mum does all my washing and gets me dressed. She says she wants to but there might be someone coming every day to help her. I don't know who that is. Mum says I might not be able to lie in some days when this person comes, and that I will have to go to bed early.'


## AGED 15 YEARS

'My brother had DMD and I saw what was happening to him, how he couldn't walk anymore and had to use a wheelchair. I've got DMD too, and I suppose for me it was just something that happened in our family. My cousin has it as well. My brother went through everything in front of me and I could see what was going to happen to me. Mum and Dad have been brilliant because they think there's nothing we cannot do. I go to the same mainstream school my brother went to so the staff are very good and know what to do, and what I need. I am about to leave school now which was the time my brother died. I don't want to think about it, but I don't know what is going to happen really. I have a Bi-pap which my brother never had. So I understand that things may be different for me.

I miss my brother. I use some of his equipment, so it feels a bit strange, him not being here, and all of his stuff which I now have. I don't want to think about it really, but at night I wonder where he is.

I am being asked to think about what I want to do after school, maybe a course or a degree. I don't know what it will be, I'm looking at options. It will need to be something not too far away from home though because I will need to live at home for help with everything. Someone told me that he couldn't do some courses because the buildings had steps and there wasn't wheelchair access. Also that the toilets were too small to have a carer in with him, even though they were supposed to be disabled toilets. So that might limit me in choices for courses.

My powered chair is good when it works but it broke down last week. I didn't have another chair. I had to sit on my bed for a day and a half whilst the emergency repair was carried out. My Mum had to stay in with me for a bit, and my Dad too when Mum had a meeting she had to go to for work. It just seemed a waste of time really, sitting about. Last time my chair broke the (children's) hospice lent me an ordinary (self propelling) chair. But this time when we phoned it was being lent to someone else.

Things I like doing? I used to like painting and drawing. I was good at it. I can't do that now really. It just gets messy because I have tried. I like computer games. The OT got a new control, a joy stick, for that. I like TV. I go to rugby matches with my Dad which are great. We get to sit at the front. We went on holiday this year to Spain, and it was great. I got to it on the beach, on the sand, and I could go down to the beach in my chair. It was a special hotel Mum had found. There were some other people in wheelchairs, and there was equipment in the rooms – a shower chair and ride in shower, and a hoist too. We had a balcony and could see the sea. I got a tan too! I want to go away again.'

## AGED 18 YEARS

'I knew I had DMD when I was 8 years old. It was when all of my family had to all go together to see the geneticist, to find out who else in the family might have DMD, but it was only me. I didn't know what it was, not until later and I was a bit older when there was something on the TV about it and I thought is that what I have got? It was scary and I was really upset.

I remember falling a lot and banging my head when I fell. I remember my friends always having to pick me up. I didn't mind so much at school, all the falling over but couldn't understand why I was falling, and trying to play football which I loved was really difficult. I used to get worried about falling down when I was out with my Mum, or just on the street. I can't remember when my wheelchair arrived; it was just there in the background somehow. I could use it when I got tired, and then I began to use it more and more. I suppose I could feel myself deteriorating really. I tried to use my rollater to walk for as long as I could.

After my mainstream primary school I went to a special school which was adapted throughout. There were lots of people in wheelchairs. It was all on the flat and there was OT and Physio there. Everyone travelled in and it was hard to see friends because everyone lived so far apart. Not like primary school where everyone was local. I met other boys with DMD and for some their condition had progressed more than mine. Some of them I got to know died in secondary school. That was very hard because they were young and died, and also because it was what I had.

It was the physio who answered my questions of what is happening to my muscles and what I could expect to be able to do. When you are young you really don't want to talk about your feelings, or ask other lads about the condition and how they manage. You just keep it all bottled up, all inside you really. It's a part of growing up I suppose that you just don't want to talk about it. I suppose it does get a bit much but I didn't really know another way.

I was aware too that I was changing shape when I was in a wheelchair and gradually lost muscle power. I had always been a slim lanky boy but I filled out and became heavy. I couldn't change that. I know some boys are skinny, but I was one of the ones that fills out. At one point I was on steroids too and that made it worse. In fact my Mum said it also made me aggressive too and very argumentative. So I came off them and settled down, it was much better for both of us. I have noticed that my circulation isn't very good and I get cold easily now.

I remember seeing the geneticist in my early teens and discussing how long I would live. That was hard, and he said that it was all only approximate and that nothing was ever hard and fast really. I did find that difficult. He was doing his job really.

Thinking back to when I first saw an OT it was at my secondary school. She introduced cutlery to me, and linked in with Social Services for things in the home. At my school the physios did all the wheelchairs. The IT teacher was the one to help with keyboard and PCs too. When I could no longer push myself in the wheelchair I was told it was time for me to get a powered chair. I had to be assessed by a technical officer who came out to see me and to determine how far I could push myself. He was very strict. It seems he didn't really believe me. I used to get so tired pushing as well. I don't know if he knew about DMD.

I was off my feet. Then when I was to get my chair I was on a waiting list for 6 months. That was so hard because I needed others to push me, as I didn't have the strength. Why did I have to wait so long at that stage? I don't understand that. I was told I was in a queue and had to wait. Then when I did get my powered chair I was told that the manual one had to be returned. That didn't make sense either really because the light one could fold up and was easy to take and the electric one couldn't go into the car until that was changed too. Even now if there is a problem with my power chair I don't have an alternative. I can't move. I don't think people understand how dependent you become on a wheelchair.

When the Social Services OT came to the home the first time it was for a ramp. My little sister was a baby and Mum had her in a buggy. The OT was insistent on a ramp starting right at the kitchen door and sloping straight away. Mum said she couldn't shut the door and have a baby in a buggy too with a ramp like that. It was dangerous. The ramp would have started from inside the door. The OT told my mother, 'Your son's disabled not you.' Well I remember that because Mum was so cross. She was always doing her best for me, fighting for things I was entitled to. The OT was not thinking about me as part of a family, just what I needed. We got a ramp but a different one, and with a different OT as well.

Then another Social Services OT came out and said I would really need a bathroom and bedroom extension on the house. That was a good idea. But it took years. There were different dates for different budgets to be passed. It was exhausting. Some work would be done then all stop. Mum spent a long time trying to find out who was responsible, and who to contact about the work, and what was happening. No one seemed to know. During that time we had four different OTs as they left after a while. It just seemed to take forever. My Mum was physically exhausted and had a breakdown from all the stress. She couldn't go to work, and she used to love her work. The extension wasn't big, a bedroom with attached bathroom and overhead hoist. The OT got an advisor in from the Muscular Dystrophy Campaign which was great, but when things went in they were different. They weren't the things which were recommended. Social Services cut corners all along. Also the people who were putting the things in didn't seem to be very well informed. The sink which can go up and down (Astor Bannerman sink for accommodating heights of chairs) had been tiled above and below and couldn't move. So we couldn't use it properly as it is at a fixed height that they put it in at.

I did recently hear from another family though of how the OT was proposing a Portacabin in the garden for their son as a bedroom. They were really annoyed. The idea was that their son would go into the garden and sleep on his own in the Portacabin at night.

We have had very different OTs and Social Workers. At the moment there isn't an OT so the Social Worker says he will cover both for us. I am not sure how well that works. Mum has had to put up with some stroppy and cross people from Social Services. It has felt as if everything has been a battle, and has had to be fought for. I don't know why this has to be. Things are difficult already, why would someone want to make it more difficult? I don't think they think fully about what they are saying to us. It used to be that the OT would check up from time to time but that does not happen now.' (Referral and request actioned and the file closed as procedure in Social Services, no longer are people reviewed regularly.)

## AGED 27 YEARS

'I am in my late twenties. I live at home with my Mum, and I employ two carers who come in daily to get me up, and put me to bed, and sort out all my personal care. I know them well and they know me so it works well. I have a part-time voluntary job which I enjoy very much and it gets me out. I am planning my summer holidays abroad this year. I have a new "tilt-in-space" chair which has been great. It means that I can take the pressure off and tilt back. I think it's good for my circulation. Also I get tired more easily now and all I have to do is tilt my chair back and have a break. It's great. It doesn't

have lights on for going out in the dark, in the winter afternoons or at night
though. I was told the NHS doesn't stretch to that.

I have had quite a few friends who have died, and it makes me think, take
life as it comes. That's all I can do. I keep fit and look after myself. I go out,
and watch football matches, and carry on with my work. I see younger lads at
the children's hospice I go to now and then. I really get so much support there.
They know what I am going through. They know how to help, and there is
always someone if I want to talk. I see the younger lads there but they don't
ask me about DMD. My chair perhaps, but not about how I am managing. I
can understand that. I never asked anyone older either. I just looked at them.
You don't ask things like that when you are younger. Now if anyone asks me
I am happy to talk about it and answer any questions.

The hospice has been so good in lots of ways, having the physio, the OT and
the Social Worker all there and getting onto services for us. That has been
great for Mum, and me. They take the hassle and get on until it's done. In fact
I would say that over the years the hospice and the staff have kept me going
really. Without them I think I would have given up long ago. It's too much on
your own really. Now I just have to get on with it and enjoy my life.'

There are several key points here, the main being that the person, whether
child, adolescent or young adult, should always be listened to.
Reproduced by permission of Daniel Morrison

## STUDY QUESTIONS

- It would be too easy to identify the key points for you. Please read through
  these accounts again, one at a time, and identify what matters to the person
  in each account.
- From the points that you have identified, and 'listened' to, consider ways in
  which the concerns could be addressed. Within these, identify the role of
  the occupational therapist.

# 5 Personal Activities of Daily Living

ALEX HOWARTH, RUTH JOHNSTON,
HEATHER McANDREW AND NICOLA TRAYNOR

## INTRODUCTION

Loss of function in personal-care activities is a constant and stark reminder of the progression of Duchenne muscular dystrophy confronting both the young person and their family in various ways on a daily basis. It is time-consuming and physically demanding for all involved but, for the young person who is dependent on others for the most intimate and basic of needs, dignity and sense of privacy are also at stake. The implications of individual beliefs, social practice and cultural diversity must be considered. Attitudes towards independence, acceptable support strategies and personal-care practices can vary enormously. Without cultural competence, therapy intervention can be construed as offensive and ineffective because of conflict with the values of the young person, their family and their community (Cronin, 2001; Awaad, 2003). For all these reasons, personal care is an area that needs to be addressed with the utmost sensitivity. Forward planning is also vital to ensure that the young person's and their family's changing needs are provided for in a timely manner.

In the first stages of loss of function, small independence aids may be useful in maintaining independent self-care skills. As the condition progresses, these aids become more difficult to use and personal-care tasks a more passive experience for the young person. The carers, who are often parents, are required to assume an increasingly active role. This can cause a strain on the parent/child relationship, as the parent is required to return to attending to their child's personal-care needs at an age at which this would not be the usual expectation. It may therefore be appropriate to seek support, where available, from community-care services to provide assistance in this area.

# GENERAL UPPER-LIMB FUNCTION FOR SELF-CARE TASKS

When considering self-care tasks, it is essential to discuss upper-limb function, as this is crucial for independence in this area.

## MOBILE ARM SUPPORTS

The pattern of progression of muscle weakness in Duchenne muscular dystrophy moves from the centre of the body outwards. This results in boys' maintaining good fine-motor skills for some time after they are unable to move their arms easily from the shoulder or against gravity. Arm supports can help to maintain independence in fine-motor tasks and a functional range of upperlimb movement for a boy with Duchenne muscular dystrophy. There are two main types of arm support: those that facilitate movement at a fixed height in a horizontal plane and the Neater Arm support, which facilitates movement in both a horizontal and a vertical plane, as controlled by the user with a switch.

The 'horizontal-only' arm supports generally consist of a clamp system to fix the support to a surface or wheelchair, a series of bars joined with moveable joints and a 'gutter'-type cushioned arm rest. The user then rests their arm (straps could be used in addition) on the support and movement is facilitated from side to side at the set height.

These arm supports can be useful in a situation in which the user is working at a stationary work surface or table for a prolonged period of time, such as when using a keyboard, writing, painting, etc. The height of this type of arm support is critical in relation to the height of the wheelchair, work surface and task at hand for it to be effective; however, it is successful in combating the effects of gravity.

The Neater Arm support also facilitates smooth vertical movement against gravity, allowing the user to maintain the ability to lift his arm from resting height to above-shoulder height as far as his passive range of movement will allow. Activities which involve lifting the arm, such as eating, brushing their teeth, scratching their nose and raising their hand in class can therefore still be carried out independently. This arm support was jointly developed by engineers from Bath Institute of Mechanical Engineering (BIME) and Cambridge University, along with the Muscular Dystrophy Campaign. The arm support consists of a metal-framed, adjustable fabric cradle for supporting the forearm. The cradle is then attached by means of a series of metal bars and frictionless joints to a vertical column. This column can either fit onto the user's powered wheelchair, powered by the wheelchair battery or onto its own free-standing base, powered by a separate battery. For powered-wheelchair users, optimal functional gains would usually be made by mounting it on their wheelchair, as the user's arm can rest in the cradle consistently and the arm support is ready to use as required. The Muscular Dystrophy Campaign (MDC) have a factsheet on mobile arm supports, which can be found on their website (*www.muscular-dystrophy.org*) or be requested by phoning 020 7720 8055 (MDC info and advice line). In addition to this factsheet, there is also a questionnaire to help determine whether a Neater Arm support is suitable for the user and their wheelchair and a justification document to help when requesting funding for the Neater Arm support.

Arm supports in general are likely to be most useful to boys with Duchenne muscular dystrophy when shoulder girdle weakness prevents them from lifting their arms or moving them easily. However, they become reliant on the support of their forearms to maintain an upright posture, as the moving surface of an arm support is likely to be too unstable for them to feel posturally secure.

For more information on either type of arm support, contact the Muscular Dystrophy Campaign.

# TOILETING

Please refer to Chapter 12 for guidelines on building requirements in relation to toileting and Chapter 8 for specific advice regarding toileting adaptations at school.

## URINE PRODUCTS

There are a variety of products that can facilitate longer-lasting independence and reduce the need for toilet transfers to pass urine as the individual's mobility reduces. The following are some examples. Each method should be considered in relation to the young person's and carer's specific situation and individual needs.

### Uridome sheath

An assessment by a suitably trained nurse will be required for this method of continence management, as the sheath has to fit precisely on the user's penis in order to prevent leakage.

### Uribag®

This device is a combination of a rigid tube with a flexible and detachable latex bag which can be folded into the tube when empty for portability. This is easily and discretely carried by the individual, in their pocket, for example. There is a cap which closes over the tube once used to seal the device until it can be emptied. Once emptied, it can be washed and reused (*www.uribag. com/uribag.php*).


**P-Bag**

The P-Bag is a discreet, portable, disposable pouch containing crystals which turn liquid into gel. It holds up to one pint of liquid before needing to be replaced. The cost implications of this should be considered, but it may be a convenient option for outings and holidays. Other similar products may be available (*www.minipotti.co.uk*).


**Urine bottle**

Urine bottles are perhaps more readily available than the above options and may be provided through the NHS (e.g. district nurse). The young person may wish to carry his own bottle, which can be rinsed following use and stored in a shoe bag or similar. The bottle will require to be sterilised at home.

Disposable bottles for single use are also available but, as with the P-Bag above, are more expensive and less eco-friendly. Furthermore, hygienic disposal may be an issue in public facilities.


*Method of use*

The bottle/bag can be used while seated in a wheelchair by adopting the following method:

• Slide the young person's bottom forward in the wheelchair.
• Move the foot rests out to the side of the wheelchair.
• Abduct the legs to each side of the wheelchair.
• Pull down the trousers and underwear at the front. Loose-fitting jogging trousers and boxer shorts are best.
• Position the bottle/bag for use.

Some boys may have their own variations of this method. Sometimes, the bottle works best in the reverse position in order to prevent urine flowing back towards the user.

It should be recognised that some boys may still prefer to use the toilet. Please refer to the following section for information regarding toilet transfers and equipment.


BOWELS

The young person will be required to transfer onto the toilet or commode for bowel movements. At present, there is no alternative method which avoids the need for transferring. It is therefore necessary to hoist the young person when they become wheelchair-dependent. Supportive equipment for sitting on the toilet is also necessary to allow him to relax and open his bowels.

Many boys suffer from constipation due to immobility, self-limited diet and slowing of peristaltic movement. This, combined with the methods required to use the toilet, can make the whole process very long indeed. It is important to be aware that it is not uncommon for young people to reduce their fluid/food intake to avoid the need to go to the toilet. A regular toileting routine can help avoid disruption, discomfort and stress, particularly in relation to the school environment.

## EQUIPMENT AND PHYSICAL ENVIRONMENT

Whilst the young person maintains the ability to carry out weight-bearing transfers, rails and a raised toilet seat or a toilet frame may be sufficient. However, as postural control deteriorates, increased support may be necessary in order to allow for a well-supported and relaxed position on the toilet. This type of support generally falls into two categories:

* support which wheels over the toilet;
* frames which fix onto the toilet itself, such as the floor-fixed MD Toilet Frame, currently available from Daily Care Ltd. This frame was specifically designed for use with a Clos-o-Mat shower toilet but can also be used with a Geberit shower toilet. It is suitable for individuals with muscular dystrophy who are non-ambulant and need to use a hoist.

For both types of support, it is important to consider the individual's specific needs, including whether lateral support, a footrest and a recline facility are necessary.

Another important consideration is whether the toilet is used by others or is used only by the young person. A fixed toilet frame support may be appropriate in an en-suite bathroom designed specifically for the young person but not in the family bathroom.

Planning ahead is essential because of the cost and space involved in suitable provision. Space may need to be found to accommodate a changing table, a mobile hoist, a wheelchair, a mobile toilet frame and two carers. Standard disabled toilets are often not big enough. In a school environment, the issue of whether a disabled student should be allocated a specific toilet also needs to be considered. If equipment needs differ between pupils, this may mean that additional space is needed to store all the equipment. As the toileting process for non-ambulant pupils can be lengthy, there is also the issue of the toilet being occupied when required by another user. For specific recommendations and details regarding toilet adaptations, please refer to Chapters 8 and 12, and the *Adaptations Manual* (Harpin, 2000).

HOISTS AND SLINGS

Two main types of hoist are available: mobile and tracking hoists. Mobile hoists are self-contained and can be used in any area of the house where space and suitable flooring allow. Tracking hoists are ceiling or wall-mounted, with a fixed route, such as bedroom to bathroom. Significant structural considerations are necessary and advice is required from structural engineers for this type of hoist. Provision of hoists may differ, depending on local policy, with the main providers being the health and social work services for use in the home.

Slings need careful assessment and vary widely between manufacturers. Most manufacturers will custom-design slings if a standard sling is not suitable. Some slings can be used with a range of hoists but this should always be clarified with the manufacturer. Slings should be reviewed regularly for fit, safety and comfort. Head support is of particular concern when assessing slings for a young person with Duchenne muscular dystrophy. Slings with semi-rigid neck and head support work well particularly as neck muscles weaken or following spinal surgery. An internal supportive chest strap may also be beneficial. Slings designed specifically for toileting are available but may not provide an adequate level of support in the longer term. As the hoisting procedure consumes both time and energy and can cause significant discomfort for the young person, some may choose to remain sitting on their sling in their wheelchair during the day. This is generally not considered to be best practice, but may be the young person's/carer's choice or preference. If this is the case, particular attention should be paid to factors that affect skin integrity issues, such as the breathability of the fabric and avoidance of increased pressure points caused by creases in the sling.

## WASHING

In the initial stages, small items of equipment, such as bath board and shower aids, may be sufficient to provide independence in this area. As the need for support and assistance with mobility increases, longer-term solutions will need to be explored, such as use of a bath as opposed to a shower.

If a bath is the preferred option, provision of a hoist (preferably ceiling track) will be necessary, as well as support within the bath itself. There are various pieces of bathing equipment available which provide differing amounts of postural support. In addition, various specialist baths with integral support devices are available on the market and these reduce the need for supplementary items of equipment.

If a shower is chosen, installation of a wet floor shower together with specialist shower chairs with adequate postural support should be investigated.

'Body dryers' may also be worth investigating, as they reduce the degree of dependence on the carer and increase the privacy and sense of dignity for the young person. Adequate heating in the bathroom is also vital to ensure that the immobile young person does not get too cold whilst being undressed/dressed, dried and transferred.

## GROOMING

With the progressive deterioration of upper-limb function, it becomes increasingly difficult for the young person to raise his arms/hands above his head.

Some small pieces of equipment are designed to facilitate this action for grooming tasks, such as a long-handled brush/comb, which require minimal movement. Consideration should be paid to the design features of items of equipment for shaving, combing hair and cleaning teeth, including weight and the type of grip. For grooming tasks normally carried out at the basin, access for a wheelchair to fit underneath (i.e. without a vanity unit, or wall-mounted) together with support for the elbows at each side of the sink is necessary. Specific recommendations regarding sink specifications are available in the *Adaptations Manual* (Harpin, 2000).

## DRESSING

In a child's early years, it is unlikely that specialist equipment will be required. For postural stability, balance and energy conservation, a seated position with feet firmly on the floor can be helpful for dressing/undressing.

As upper-limb function diminishes, the amount of assistance required increases and small items of equipment such as a dressing stick may prove useful.

Choice of clothing can also have a significant impact. Clothing should be comfortable and easy to get on and off: loose, with big head opening and minimal fastenings. A few UK companies and several US companies specialise in providing a range of clothing, sportswear and outdoor wear adapted to the needs of wheelchair users. Garments are usually a bit more expensive than their standard alternative but the adaptations may make life easier in small ways and may also help with larger issues, such as transfers, skin integrity, toileting/continence care and independence in dressing.

Adapted trousers are usually shaped in specific ways to be more comfortable and better-fitting in a seated position than standard trousers. Trouser legs will be longer so they do not creep up the leg when sitting and are often roomier to allow access to leg bags or orthoses. The back of the trousers will be high-rise and the front may be lower so that the waistband remains at waist height when sitting.

Materials are usually designed to be breathable, comfortable and non-abrasive. Seams should be designed carefully not to coincide with pressure points. Pockets are often designed vertically to prevent items falling out and belt loops can be strengthened to help with pulling the trousers on. Zips can be made longer to allow easier access for toileting and various sorts of fastenings can be considered, such as Velcro™, poppers and hooks. Smaller Velcro™ fastenings can be easier for people with Duchenne muscular dystrophy, as they require less strength than large areas of Velcro™. Trousers can be purchased with side as well as front openings and can be designed with front flaps (like sailor-style trousers) to minimise fastenings whilst maximising privacy.

Jackets can be designed to be shorter at the front to allow a better fit when sitting, or backless to allow for moulded seating. Ponchos and capes can be used as alternatives to jackets. Various types of leg covers are also available similar to short sleeping bags but less bulky and available in a variety of materials to allow for different weather conditions and seasons.

Some companies will adapt clothing to particular needs but it may also be possible to design specific clothing with the help of a local seamstress.

## EASY REACHER

Although not related to any specific area of self-care, a difficulty that can arise for the individual who has difficulty with postural control is reaching for or picking up items beyond their immediate reach. For the young person with muscular dystrophy who has reduced proximal stability and reduced power in upper limbs, this may indeed be a problem. It is important to remember that there are pieces of equipment available which can assist with this, such as a 'grab stick'/'easy reacher'. This eliminates the need to move beyond the base of support when trying to pick up objects. In addition, some chairs/wheelchairs swivel on their base to allow the individual to turn round to reach items rather than having to twist.

## EATING

The activity of eating or feeding is one which, by its very nature, involves upper-limb function. Cutlery and cups are held and manipulated by the hands and, once loaded, are lifted to the mouth. For the individual with muscular dystrophy, this basic survival task becomes very demanding as muscle weakness progresses, grip strength becomes poor and it becomes increasingly difficult to lift the hands/arms against gravity.

It therefore becomes necessary to explore alternative methods of eating and drinking using small pieces of equipment that are available. Initially, lightweight cutlery with chunky handles may be beneficial as it reduces the weight to be lifted to the mouth and facilitates an easier grip. Other alternatives such as elevating the plate height, rocker knives and angled cutlery will minimize the amount of active arm, wrist and hand movement required (Disabled Living Foundation, 2005).

Plate guards or high-rimmed plates may help to prevent food falling off the plate and assist in loading a fork or spoon.

For drinking, there are various types of cups/mugs/bottles which may be easier for the individual to use independently. Sports bottles can be useful, as they are less likely to spill and may be more aesthetically acceptable though when full may be too heavy. Lightweight cups and mugs may also be beneficial to accommodate reduced power, but it is important to ensure that these are easy to grip – it may be necessary to have two handles.

As the upper limbs become increasingly weak, the individual may lean his head forward to meet his hands, thus compensating for being unable to lift his hands fully up towards his face. At this stage, it may be useful to explore the use of long straws that have non-return valves for drinking, such as Pat Saunders Drinking Straws, thus eliminating the need to lift the cup to the mouth (Chester et al., 2001). It may also be beneficial to raise the height of the table to axilla height, to support the elbows and forearms and reduce the distance to be lifted to reach the face (Wilsdon, 1998). It is important to note, however, that once a young person has had spinal surgery, he may no longer be able to use this compensatory method of leaning the head forward to meet the hands (Harpin et al., 2002).

As the individual becomes less able to lift cutlery and cups to his face for independent feeding, it may be necessary to explore equipment that provides support to the forearm to facilitate this movement, such as mobile arm supports (see above). For eating and drinking, those which enable movement in both the horizontal and vertical planes are necessary to facilitate lifting to the face. Another option at this stage is to explore equipment that carries out the movement for you, such as the Neater Eater. The Neater Eater clamps to the table and consists of a board and an extended 'arm' which has an attachment for the spoon/fork. This can be moved by a variety of methods, depending on the user's specific needs (Chester et al., 2001). For those with Duchenne muscular dystrophy, the types which are most likely to be beneficial either have a lever action where the 'arm' is moved using a smaller lever close to the individual or the powered version which is operated by switches or a joystick (*www.neater.co.uk*).

The same company that manufactures the Neater Eater and mobile arm support (Neater Solutions) also provides the Neater Snacker, which is an extended 'arm' which is clamped to the side of a table and can be angled as required. It has a sandwich holder at the end of the arm which can secure a variety of snacks (sandwiches, pizzas, etc.). For this piece of equipment to be used, however, it needs to be set up, loaded and angled for the user and therefore involves a higher degree of dependency (*www.neater.co.uk*).

## SLEEPING

Just as good daytime positioning is of paramount importance for the young person with Duchenne muscular dystrophy, so is night-time positioning for sleep. Once pelvic instability is apparent, a postural management plan should be developed to promote optimum posture. This is essential to minimise the risks of deformity, such as the limitations of movement and pain caused by joint contractures or spinal curvatures that impact upon lung capacity and respiratory function.

When addressing the management of posture with the young person, parents and carers, it is very important to try to achieve a balance in the discussion and not create unrealistic expectations about the prevention of deformity (which is inevitable in light of progressive muscle weakness and loss of movement) but also not to induce a sense of helplessness and a disregard for the importance of postural care. It is important that all those involved with the young person understand that the risk of deformity is high and is, to a certain extent, unavoidable, but that much can be done to help to minimise the extent of and reduce the effects of deformity.

The young person's postural needs must be managed throughout their daily lives which includes overnight positioning. A 24-hour postural management programme should be developed to address the sitting, standing and lying positions that the young person will need. This programme should be designed in conjunction with the young person, their carer, their occupational therapist and their physiotherapist. The aims of the positioning programme should ideally be formally documented along with guidelines for positioning the young person correctly. The young person's postural needs will require regular review and the postural management programme will require to be adjusted accordingly.

In the management of lying positions for sleep, initially, advice on symmetrical positioning in bed and postural supports to help with this are likely to be sufficient. The use of firm cushions and rolls can provide adequate support to maintain a good lying posture for sleep and have the added benefit of being easily positioned and removed. In the early stages of the condition, the young person may be able to help to position and remove the supports. The disadvantage of this type of postural control is that the supports may move out of position during sleep.

A variety of beds are available which are known as 'profiling beds'. These beds are electrically powered and are composed of a platform with three or four separate sections which can be moved independently of one another, allowing for a position to be achieved other than flat lying; for example, the head and feet may be raised, or the head raised and the feet lowered. A profiling bed may be useful as part of a postural management positioning programme and it could also allow the young person a degree of independence in altering their position in bed and sitting up.

Profiling beds also allow the height of the bed from the floor to be adjusted and this can be useful to the young person in the early stage of the condition: a higher surface requires less muscle power to stand up from, as the legs can be lowered to the floor in a straight-leg position, rather than trying to rise against gravity from a flexed-knee position. Bed-height adjustment is also helpful if the young person is able to manage to side transfers on/off the bed using a transfer board. Carers will also find the ability to raise the bed to an optimum-working height invaluable for transfers, helping with dressing, carrying out stretches or helping the young person to move. The risk of back strain is then minimised.

As the condition progresses, it may be necessary to provide an increased level of support to manage the young person's lying posture effectively. At this stage, a sleep system is worth considering. The aim of a sleep system is to combine symmetrical positioning with a comfortable and supportive position for sleep. Sleep systems are often supplied by the same manufacturers as seating systems and there are various different designs available, in terms of both structure and material. Some consist of a base with brackets and cushions that can be attached to support the individual in a variety of positions. Other sleep systems consist of a mattress overlay that can be moulded, by the positioning of padded supports, to provide contoured all-round body support.

For any sleep system, an assessment is required to create an individually customised combination of supports. Suppliers will normally provide a free assessment and some may offer to loan the system out for a few nights' trial by prior arrangement. This is invaluable in the process of determining which particular system suits the needs of both the young person and their carers; some sleep systems are easier to adjust than others; some are more compatible with pressure-reducing mattresses or profiling beds. Follow-up support from the supplier is also a consideration.

## CALL SYSTEMS

When the young person is dependent on a powered wheelchair for mobility and has reduced ability to adjust their own posture, they will often rely heavily on parents and carers to make postural adjustments for them. These adjustments are of the sort that able-bodied people take for granted, such as shifting weight when sitting, to relieve pressure areas. This need to change position can also occur when lying in bed. This can be alleviated by the use of a pressure-relieving mattress, which will automatically relieve pressure points, along with a profiling bed (see above), which can be adjusted by the young person through the use of a remote handset.

Even with these measures in place, the young person is likely to still need the small adjustments that only a carer can make for them and it is crucial that they (and their carers) should be reassured by easy contact during the night. It is often the case in a two-storey house that the carers will be sleeping on a different floor from the young person and this makes it very difficult for the young person to call for help during the night. A call system should be put in place which can be easily operated by the young person and alerts the carer to their needs. This could be a monitor such as those used for babies, a walkie-talkie system or a remotely controlled doorbell. In some cases, the existing phone system could be used to make internal calls if there is an extension in each room.

The choice of call system would depend on the upper-limb function of the young person, the ease with which it could be sited on their bed for use and the individual circumstances of the family (e.g. if the carers to be called on have a young baby sharing their room or wish only one of them to be roused, a noisy call system could be replaced by the sort of vibrating system used by people who are hearing-impaired).

Remote doorbell systems can be fairly easily converted for use with switches activated by only the lightest of touches or by parts of the body other than the hand. Local bioengineering staff should be able to help with this and could probably suggest other possible solutions.


## SEXUAL HEALTH AND WELL-BEING

Sexuality is fundamental to an individual's health and well-being, irrespective of whether a disability is involved. For boys with Duchenne muscular dystrophy, the onset of adolescence has usually been preceded by a significant loss of mobility and independence. Whilst function in activities of daily living is addressed, sexual issues are often overlooked or ignored at this crucial stage in the development of sexual awareness and experience. Boys with Duchenne muscular dystrophy, like all other disabled people, need to be recognised as sexual beings, with sexual and emotional needs and desires.

Their sexual health and well-being cannot be ignored, but the extent to which it falls within the remit of occupational therapy is a matter for debate, on both a professional and a personal level. It may be that the occupational therapist plays a key role, perhaps because of the relationship established with the young person, family and carers; or because of historical or pragmatic reasons within a particular multidisciplinary setting; or because of specialist knowledge and experience. On the other hand, the occupational therapist may feel reluctant to take on this role, on the grounds of personal inhibition, cultural background or lack of expertise and training.

Disabled people and their family and carers should be able to access full information, advice and support on areas of sexual health that are relevant to their specific needs and, whatever the level of intervention provided by the occupational therapist, it is essential that he/she is aware of appropriate resources. Some organisations such as Relate provide a service for everyone who needs help and advice with regard to relationships, whilst others specialise in helping disabled people. For example, although the Association to Aid the Sexual and Personal Relationships of People with a Disability (SPOD) no longer exists an organisation called Outsiders has recently taken over some of its roles, including its helpline. Outsiders was originally founded in 1979 and is an independent, nationwide group run by and for disabled people. It provides the opportunity for group members to communicate and meet up in order to gain confidence in socialising, make new friends and find partners; receive support throughout the process both on a one-to-one basis or through group work; and to access information including advice sheets, a list of relevant books and an in-house publication called *Practical Tips*. The Proud Consortium, in conjunction with Contact a Family, has also recently published a series of booklets to support young disabled people, their parents/carers and teachers with regard to sex and relationships. These booklets (referenced in the bibliography at the end of this book) contain very useful advice and resource information.

## KEY POINTS

- It is crucial that occupational therapists have an appreciation of cultural differences and values when addressing this sensitive and personal area to protect the young person's dignity.
- Occupational therapists, when making recommendations in relation to personal-care issues, have to be aware not only of the equipment and the resources available, but also of current policies and procedures, for example, on moving and handling and child protection.
- Many self-care activities rely on upper-limb function/movement. Various small pieces of equipment may be beneficial initially; however, in the longer term, the use of mobile arm supports should be explored to maintain functional independence.
- Occupational therapists should at least have an awareness of appropriate resources and contacts to provide the young person with muscular dystrophy support in relation to the area of sexual health and well-being.
- Consideration of profiling and height-adjustable beds and sleep systems is essential to promote 24-hour postural care, facilitate longer-lasting independence (e.g. for transfers) and accommodate moving and handling requirements.
- Forward planning is vital to ensure that the young person and their family's changing needs are provided for in a timely manner.

## CASE STUDY

Keiran is a 12-year-old boy with Duchenne muscular dystrophy. He has four siblings: an elder brother (16) who does not have Duchenne muscular dystrophy, an older sister (14), a younger sister (9) and a younger brother (18 months) with Duchenne muscular dystrophy. Keiran's parents have not been keen to take up the offer of genetic counselling and neither of Keiran's sisters has been tested to see if they carry the genetic mutation responsible for Duchenne muscular dystrophy.

The family live in a four-bedroomed, adapted house with garage, rented from a housing association. The house is purpose-built for a wheelchair user so the facilities are not specific to the needs of this family. Keiran's bedroom is on the ground floor and the bathroom is not en-suite but is also on the ground floor. The other bedrooms are on the upper floor of the house. His brother has a bedroom to himself, his sisters share and his youngest brother still sleeps in a cot in his parents' room.

Dad does not have a full-time job but picks up temporary labouring work on a regular basis. Mum is a full-time housewife. The family mostly manages on their benefit entitlement. Keiran is in his first year of secondary at the local mainstream high school.

Keiran's parents are finding it increasingly difficult to manage with the baby in their room. The baby is easily disturbed and Mum and Dad are getting very little sleep. When they do get to sleep, they are often woken by Keiran shouting upstairs, asking to have his position changed in bed and this often wakes the baby, too.

Mum and Dad have only recently begun to use the mobile hoist they have for Keiran. When Keiran has a shower, he is hoisted into his shower chair in his bedroom due to the lack of space in the bathroom and wheeled through the hall to the bathroom. Mum and Dad are finding it difficult to take him to and from the bathroom for his shower in a discrete and dignified way (the house is often busy with the children's friends). Keiran also complains about getting cold on his way to the bathroom.

Currently, the only large pieces of equipment that Keiran has are his powered wheelchair, mobile hoist, height-adjustable profiling bed and shower/toilet chair. Although Keiran would probably benefit from other equipment, his parents have been reluctant to accept further equipment until recently, as they feel that the more Keiran does for himself, the more function he will maintain.

There is limited space to extend the house, as the complex adjoins an inner-city protected nature reserve. The family already live in the largest house in the complex and the housing association, though happy to share the cost of any proposed extension/adaptation to the house with the local social work department, do not wish their property to become too specific to one family's needs, as they have to consider the long-term view of the property.

Keiran's parents are beginning to feel quite desperate and say that they are now ready to accept anything that will help Keiran. Both of them are beginning to suffer back pain and they are gradually accepting that Keiran is not maintaining function and recently has deteriorated significantly.

## STUDY QUESTIONS

• What, if any, possibilities exist to improve Keiran's access to the bathroom?
• How could Keiran alert his parents to his needs during the night and not disturb the baby?
• Is there anything that could be done to reduce the number of times that Keiran may need his position adjusted during the night?
• How could Keiran's equipment be rationalised to create space in his room?


## SOLUTION

A small extension was made from the family garage, which was then joined to the house to create a new bedroom for Keiran, provide equipment storage space and enlarge the existing bathroom. A car port was created to allow all-weather access to the car.

An additional entrance was made into the bathroom from the new bedroom, allowing Keiran more privacy when using the bathroom. The bathroom had a wet floor shower area and body dryer installed. A ceiling track hoist was fitted, running from the bedroom to the bathroom in a line which included the bed, floor space and toilet. This meant that the mobile hoist was no longer needed and this saved on space.

A switch mounted on Keiran's bed (which could be adjusted in sensitivity) was connected to a vibration pad (of the sort used by hearing-impaired people) which was then placed under the pillow of one of Keiran's parents. This allowed Keiran to alert his parents to his needs during the night without waking the baby.

Keiran was assessed for, and provided with, a pressure-relieving mattress which reduced the number of times he needed to be repositioned in the night. He was also assessed for a sleep system to support his posture when sleeping and funding was being sought for this.

Around the same time, Keiran's respiratory function was reviewed and it was suggested that he would benefit from overnight oxygen. This had a positive effect on the number of times Keiran was waking during the night. In addition, Keiran's parents moved downstairs into his old bedroom with the baby and plan to gradually move the baby into his own room upstairs.

# 6 Seating

JOY BLAKENEY AND RUTH JOHNSTON

## INTRODUCTION

The importance of appropriate seating for all children cannot be overestimated. The aims of good seating are: to achieve a good postural position; to maintain functional ability; and to ensure comfort (Harpin, 2003). Seating which promotes a good sitting posture will also promote effective upper-limb function which is essential for a variety of activities, including feeding, writing and play. In the case of the young person with Duchenne muscular dystrophy, the consideration and provision of appropriate seating are particularly important both in relation to static seating and wheelchairs. It is crucial that seating needs are considered from an early age to prevent or delay deformities and promote optimal function (Harpin et al., 2002). This should be monitored and reviewed on a regular basis to accommodate any changes as the person's condition progresses.

## CONSIDERATIONS

There are many factors to take into account when assessing the seating needs of young people with Duchenne muscular dystrophy. The 'Seating Assessment and Recommendations' form and examples (Appendices II, III and IV) are intended to act as a prompt and a guide for the various factors which may influence your choice of chair.

Through assessment, it is important to gain information about the individual's abilities, including his sitting balance (unsupported), pelvic stability, muscle strength, symmetry, upper-limb function, any existing deformities (e.g. spinal) or contractures and skin integrity. These factors will then help you to determine what features a suitable chair should have. For example, the individual who is still mobile but has reduced proximal stability and poor sitting balance when he tires may require a fairly basic chair with minimal support, which allows for independent transfers. However, for the individual whose condition is more advanced and is no longer mobile, you may consider a much more supportive seat with pressure-relieving cushion and padding/

supports to promote a good posture and prevent further deformities, contractures and pressure sores. At this stage, seating is likely to be in the form of a powered wheelchair to maintain the young person's mobility.

It is important to determine what the wishes, attitudes and expectations of the young person and his family are in relation to supportive seating. By determining this and taking it into account when working with them, you are more likely to achieve acceptance. Often, the appearance of the chair will be a significant consideration for the young person and his parents.

It is useful when carrying out a seating assessment to explore at least two options for suitable seating, examining the pros and cons of all possibilities and comparing these. This will avoid the temptation to choose a piece of equipment just because you are familiar with it. The 'Seating Assessment and Recommendations' form (Appendix II) therefore allows for comparision of two different chairs.

## SEAT WIDTH

When assessing the width of seat required, it is important to consider variations in clothing, such as, if the measuring takes place in summer, remember that the individual may wear thicker clothes in winter and therefore require extra space (Harpin, 2003). Some extra width may be required to enable positioning a hoist sling (Harpin, 2003). It should be recognised that it is not felt to be best practice for a hoist sling to be left in situ between hoisting. It is important that the chair provides adequate support to stabilise the pelvis, and avoid pelvic obliquity. The armrests should also be close enough to the body to avoid having to lean sideways excessively to use these (Harpin, 2003).

## SEAT DEPTH

When considering the seat depth, it is important to ensure that the spine is well supported and poor postures such as sacral sitting and posterior pelvic tilt are discouraged. Support should be maintained along the length of the femur. When the hips are against the seat back, there should be a gap of one to two inches between the back of the knees and the seat upholstery (Harpin, 2003). This ensures that nerves and blood vessels running behind the knee are not compressed, causing pins and needles or numbness and avoiding tissue trauma (USAtech, 2004).

## ADAPTATIONS

There are various different adaptations and modifications available for most chairs on the market. This allows you to 'tailor' the chair to the needs of each individual. For the young person with Duchenne muscular dystrophy, there are several adaptations which should be considered at different stages. These are listed below.

## FOOTPLATES

These are crucial, and must be considered from an early stage as it may be possible to delay or prevent plantar foot deformities (a common difficulty for young people with Duchenne muscular dystrophy). Ideally footplates should maintain a 90° angle at the ankle (Harpin et al., 2002) and should be adjustable in both height and angle, to accommodate the individual's foot/ankle position as it changes (Healthcare, 2004). If the individual is wearing an ankle–foot orthosis (AFO), this may determine the angle of the footplate. It is also useful to have split footplates to allow for these to be adjusted individually and therefore accommodate any differences between the left and right foot. Heel straps at the back of the footplate ensure that the young man's foot doesn't slip off, as, over time, the ability to move the foot reduces.

In the case of a wheelchair which is to be used outdoors, thought must be given to the height of the footplates from the ground to avoid contact with the kerb, whilst also being mindful of knee and hip position.

It is important to consider the skin integrity of the young person's feet, what type of footwear he will be wearing and thus the implications for pressure points, friction and whether the footrests themselves need to be padded (where thin or no footwear is worn). Older adolescents may prefer to wear slippers or soft shoes which accommodate foot deformities which can develop.

## PELVIC AND LATERAL/THORACIC SUPPORTS

From a young age, people with Duchenne muscular dystrophy tend to lean on one elbow (Harpin, 2003) when seated due to the deterioration in trunk control and resultant difficulty in supporting an upright sitting position. This position is asymmetrical, however, and therefore should be discouraged due to the long-term implications for deformities. A symmetrical posture can be encouraged through the use of side pads. As irreversible changes occur in the spinal position, the side pads can be altered to accommodate this and control curves (Harpin, 2003).

It is important to ackowledge, however, that no individual can ever sit symmetrically all of the time, and frequent changes in position need to be encouraged.

## HEAD REST/SUPPORT

This type of support will become more important as the young person's neck control reduces. A support is also crucial following spinal surgery and will provide support to allow for change in position if using a tilt-in-space seat.

If the young person is to be transported in a vehicle while still seated in a wheelchair, it is essential that a crash-tested head rest is fitted for safety reasons.

## ARM RESTS/SUPPORTS

Arm rests support the elbows, the forearms and, indirectly, provide compensatory support to the shoulders. They should ideally be adjustable in both height and width (between arm rests), thereby providing optimal support and allowing for growth. The covering and padding of these arm rests should be suitable to provide pressure relief and comfort. They may be used as an anchor point for the elbow to facilitate movement as the shoulder girdle weakens; therefore, they should be at a height which provides support to the arms, with the shoulders in a comfortable position.

Arm rests which angle will also allow the tray angle to be altered, which may be useful in adjusting the position of books and to promote an upright sitting posture.

Sliding transfers in and out of the chair can also be facilitated where the arm rests are removable. This may be easier for the individual than attempting a transfer involving sit-to-stand (Harpin, 2003).

## SEAT BASE/CUSHIONS

It is important that the seat base is firm enough to provide adequate support for the pelvis, however pressure-relieving material is also essential to promote comfort and prevent pressure sores and deformities. Many of the specialised static seats available on the market have pressure-relieving foam integrated into the base of the seat itself and therefore avoid the need for an additional cushion. However, in the case of a wheelchair, it is necessary to identify an appropriate type of pressure relief for the seat which will usually be in the form of a pressure-relieving cushion. As the individual becomes increasingly immobile, pressure relief becomes correspondingly important.

Care should also be taken with wheelchairs to ensure that the seat base is taut and not 'sagging', as this will not provide a stable or level base to sit on or to position a cushion on (Muscular Dystrophy Campaign, 2006).

## TILT-IN-SPACE

This facility is increasingly available in specialised seating and may be appropriate for this client group to provide a change in position, and therefore reduce pressure points and increase comfort, as their independent mobility reduces.

## ADDITIONAL SUPPORTS

There are various other adaptations which can be fitted onto seating to provide extra support where the individual's postural control is deteriorating. The details of these and their availability will vary, depending on the specific chair being considered. Therefore, the following is purely a list of adaptations which may be required:

• knee pads;
• pelvic strap;
• chest strap;
• waistcoat;
• supportive harness;
• abductor pommels.

## MATERIALS

When deciding on a suitable piece of seating equipment, it is important to consider the material/fabric which covers it. As the young person is likely to be sitting in this seat/wheelchair for prolonged periods, it is important that the material is breathable and therefore more comfortable, especially during the hotter months.

The fabric should be easy to clean and it is important to identify who will take responsibility to do this regularly. Some products will have fabric that can be wiped clean, whereas others may have removable covers that can be fully washed. Spare covers are beneficial.

The durability of the material/fabric should also be considered, as specialised seats and wheelchairs are costly purchases which are expected to last well even with daily use.

Many of the companies who provide seating options will also offer a selection of colours or patterns of materials/fabric covers. The young person should be made aware of the options and given the choice, as he is more likely to feel a sense of ownership of the chair if he has been involved in the selection process, including choosing the colour.

## TABLES/TRAYS

Assessment is necessary of the table/work surface that the individual will be accessing while seated. Will he be sitting at a school desk or is a special desk or tray required?

If the individual is to use a table/desk, it is important to determine whether he can get close enough to it or requires a table with a 'cut-out' front. A cut out table may provide better support for his elbows, thus eliminating the need for forward flexion at the trunk to rest on the table. 'Cut-outs' may also be required to accommodate wheelchair fixtures such as a joystick control.

The ideal table height to promote hand function is two inches above the flexed elbows while the individual is seated (Amundson, 2001); however, for those with Duchenne muscular dystrophy, it may be beneficial to have the work surface higher, with the elbows supported. This will eliminate some of the need to work against gravity when lifting the arms up, as this becomes increasingly difficult due to reduced proximal muscle power in the upper limbs. It may therefore be most beneficial to have a height-adjustable table to achieve the optimum height. Various types of height-adjustable tables are available on the market, including electric types with hand-held controls which allow the user maximum independence. The work surface must also be wide enough to accommodate a comfortable position for the individual's elbows.

It may also be beneficial to have non-slip matting (e.g. dycem) placed on the work surface to support and stabilise the individual's elbows and forearms and prevent slipping. It is crucial, however, that attention is paid to potential shearing forces on the skin.

Depending on the amount of active movement that the individual has in his upper limbs, it may be beneficial to attach padding to the work surface to avoid increased pressure on the elbows. This should, however, be detachable, as it may impede functional movement and would only be required at specific times. A doughnut-shaped ring of tubigrip rolled in on itself several times can be useful for this, as it will support and pad the elbow but allow movement around the work surface. Sheepskin elbow pads can also be made with Velcro™ tabs to allow for attaching and removing from the table/tray easily.

To avoid moving and handling issues, it may be necessary to have a table which is on wheels to bring it into close proximity to the individual. The individual may lean on the table when rising to standing from sitting (Harpin, 2003). It is therefore important that the table is stable and that, if it is on wheels, the brakes are always applied when static. Attention should also be paid to whether there are crossbars under the table which may interfere with the young person's feet or footplates.

## WHEELCHAIRS

As the young person's condition progresses and the level of mobility reduces, it will become necessary for him to consider using a wheelchair. It must be acknowledged that the introduction of a wheelchair is a significant stage in recognition of the deterioration of the condition and is therefore highly sensitive. Initially, only a manual wheelchair may be required for use outdoors or where an increased amount of walking is involved, such as for outings. Gradually, however, it will become increasingly necessary for the individual to progress to using a powered chair for both indoors and outdoors.

The psychological impact of this process on both the child and his family, particularly the parents, should be recognised. The way this is presented to the parents should emphasise the potential benefits of using a wheelchair to the child, including increased energy levels and reduced muscle fatigue (Muscular Dystrophy Campaign, 2006).

The process involved in assessment for, and provision of, wheelchairs will vary from area to area. There are usually specific regional centres that deal purely with wheelchairs with staff who are highly specialised in this area. All of the considerations mentioned under static seating are also relevant to wheelchairs. The following provides an overview, with general advice and guidance. Other documents are available which provide in-depth information regarding all aspects of wheelchair assessment and provision, such as the *Muscular Dystrophy Campaign Wheelchair Provision for Children and Adults with Muscular Dystrophy and Other Neuromuscular Conditions: Best Practice Guidelines* (Muscular Dystrophy Campaign, 2006) and the *National Clinical Guidelines for Specialised Wheelchair Seating* (BRSM).

When the young person begins to use a wheelchair for longer periods, his body position will become increasingly static. The wheelchair, which is likely now to become his supportive seating, will have to provide the correct amount of postural support and pressure relief to reduce the risk of deformities, contractures and pressure sores/ulcers and to maximise comfort. Good postural support may also help to aid lung function through preserving the thoracic capacity. It is suggested that postural control should be introduced into the wheelchair prescription when the young person begins to use it on a daily basis (Muscular Dystrophy Campaign, 2006).

Although, at this stage, the young person's mobility has become compromised, it is important to ensure that he maintains the maximum level of independence where possible. Therefore, it is crucial that the control for the powered chair is fully accessible for the young person and can be utilised with minimal upper-limb movement and strength. It is important to note that many boys develop a scoliosis towards one side and therefore the position of their control is crucial to avoid reinforcing this. At this point, it may be necessary to consider the provision of powered mobile arm supports, attached to the wheelchair and powered by a separate battery. This will help to support the young person's forearms and promote continued use of the hands and fingers as weakness of the arm muscles increases. By providing this external forearm support, it should be possible to maintain independent function for a variety of activities involving upper-limb movement, such as independent feeding, putting hands up in class and scratching the nose.

As with static seating, other electrically operated wheelchair features, which may be necessary or beneficial, include: a reclining backrest; a seat and backrest that 'tilt-in-space'; and independently height-adjustable leg rests (Harpin et al., 2002). These features are important in providing a change in position which the individual may not be able to achieve himself. Wheelchairs are also available which move the user from a sitting position to a fully supported standing position.

The safety issues around the use of a powered wheelchair must be considered, including training that may be required for the individual. It is important to monitor and manage the speed restrictions on the chair and adjust this as appropriate, for example as the young person's steering improves. This may help to avoid damage to the chair and injury to the young person's feet or shoes.

Some powered chairs are only suitable for use indoors. If a chair is to be used outdoors, there will be further safety issues to be considered, especially going up/down kerbs and along uneven pavements/roads. If going out in the dark, reflective clothing or reflective paint may be useful. It is essential that you consult with the wheelchair providers regarding any such necessary adaptations and whether the young person would be insured to use the chair outside.

Practicalities relating to the wheelchair, such as where it can be stored when not in use, where it can be charged and whether it can be lifted in and out of the car easily, need to be considered. Where the young person is using a powered chair, the family will need to determine whether the vehicle they use can be adapted to transport the boy in his chair or whether a new adapted vehicle is required.

Access around both the home and school environments needs to be assessed when a wheelchair is to be used.

## ENVIRONMENTAL CONSIDERATIONS

### SCHOOL

As with any piece of equipment, contextual assessment of the individual's seating needs is crucial and, therefore, assessment both within school and at home is required.

If the young person requires supportive seating at school, the classroom environment and any other class or area in which the seat will be used need to be considered. Where a wheelchair is being explored, the whole school environment and access around it will need to be assessed (see Chapter 8).

When introducing supportive seating into a school, it is important that liaison takes place with the school staff and that they feel involved in the whole process. The young person's use of the supportive seating will be partly, if not entirely, dependent on school staff's assistance and it is therefore crucial that they have a good understanding of why it is required, when it should be used and how to position the young person in it for maximum function and benefit.

Unlike therapists, school staff are unlikely to be familiar with supportive seating and therefore will require guidance and reassurance with this. Ongoing liaison with the school staff will be required to ensure effective use, monitoring and evaluation of the chosen seat.

## HOME

At home, it is necessary to determine what the principle use of the seating is to be; namely is it to provide support to engage in activity or is it for relaxation? Once this is established and the location in which the chair is to be used is determined, it is important to consider environmental factors, such as space limitations, family expectations and height/size of dining table in situ, if it is to be used at the dining table.

In the early stages, while the young person is still mobile, he may only require a supportive static seat at home for use while engaging in tabletop activities, such as eating. However, as the condition progresses and mobility deteriorates, the individual is likely to use an electric wheelchair during the day and it may also be appropriate to have an 'easy chair' or supportive recliner for relaxation and comfort at home. This will provide a change of position from the wheelchair and many of these are now multi-adjustable, electrically operated, wheeled and supportive. Some offer the facility to raise and lower the legs and it may be possible to have arm rests which lift out of the way to allow for side transfers (Harpin, 2003). A reclining back rest is important to allow for a change in position and relieve pressure. For many families, it is important that home seating is aesthetically pleasing and 'fits in' with their current furniture. This should be taken into account as much as possible. Some companies may offer the option of users providing their own material.

## EMPLOYMENT

Considering the young person with Duchenne muscular dystrophy who may move on to employment, a powered office-style chair is available which was specifically designed for this client group. The eMove powered chair has the following features: powered rise; powered seat tilt; arm rests and footplates rise with the seat; adjustable back rest and seat; optional head rest; tight turning circle; narrow width; joystick control; and swing-back arm rests (Harpin, 2003; eMove, 2007).

## FUNDING

Sources of funding for pieces of equipment will vary from area to area and advice should be sought locally. However, in general, the local education authority will fund equipment for school, such as a specialist static chair. Static seating for home, however, is usually funded by the local social work department. All agencies involved in the provision of seating equipment are likely to have set criteria and may have agreed contracts with specific companies which will influence which chair is provided.

In relation to wheelchairs, in general, these are provided by specific centres and funded by the local health authority. However, there may again be variations between areas and specific criteria for provision of different types of wheelchairs.

In the event that an individual or his family want a piece of seating equipment or a specific wheelchair that will not be provided by the statutory organisations (Health and Social Work), funding may be sought from other sources, such as charitable organisations. In individual cases, the statutory body may agree to fund the desired equipment to the cost of its statutory equivalent.

## SERVICING

When assessing for and providing specialist seating, it is essential to consider the servicing requirements and general insurance for the chair. Each company will have their own recommendations; however, it is important that the responsibility for servicing is adopted by someone for seating provided both at home and at school.

## CAR SEATING

A booster seat and diagonal three-point harness will not provide adequate support for the young person who is no longer able to maintain a symmetrical posture against the forces of gravity when travelling in the car. It is therefore necessary to explore alternatives which provide extra support. Some specialised car seats are available which are suitable for children and teenagers, and provide the required level of support. The limit to these car seats is determined according to the weight of the young person and should be checked in the manufacturer's guidelines. It should be noted, however, that transfers into these can be difficult. Adaptations to cars are sometimes possible and can include swivel seating (Adaptacar, 2004). Advice can be sought from a paediatric occupational therapist regarding specific car seats. Your local driving assessment centre may offer passenger assessments to help with this.

Guidance on the safe transportation of wheelchairs is provided by the Medical Devices Agency (2005).

# KEY POINTS

- It is essential that the young person and his parents are consulted throughout the process of choosing supportive seating, as this will result in a sense of ownership and increased compliance.
- Liaison with and training of education staff are crucial in improving the effectiveness of and compliance with specialised seating within school.
- A good sitting posture is important for all children and helps to promote hand function for a variety of activities, including feeding, writing and play.
- Good postural support can help to prevent or delay contractures and deformities and aid lung function through preserving thoracic capacity.
- There are several aspects involved in the assessment for specialised seating, including seat height, width and depth, arm rests, footplates and head rest. The 'Seating Assessment and Recommendations' form (Appendix II) gives prompts regarding these areas.
- As the individual becomes more immobile, pressure relief, possibly in the form of a pressure cushion, becomes increasingly important.
- Tilt-in-space facilities in a chair as well as independently adjustable back rests and footrests facilitate a change in position for an individual who may be unable to achieve this himself.
- A wheelchair will become necessary as the young person's mobility reduces and will gradually be required for use both indoors and outdoors. It is important to emphasise the positive gains of this to the young person and his family, including increased energy levels.
- An 'easy chair' or supportive recliner may be beneficial at home to provide an opportunity for relaxation, comfort and a change of position for the young person.

# CASE STUDY

John is an eight-year-old boy with Duchenne muscular dystrophy. He lives with his mother, brother and sister in a two-storey council house. Mum is a single parent, his brother is four years older and his sister is five years younger than he is. John gets on well with his brother and sister and wants to be as active as them.

John's mobility is beginning to deteriorate; he is beginning to fall more frequently and experiences difficulties with climbing stairs. Although, at present, John uses a 'normal' chair at home and school, he is becoming less stable when standing and sitting.

John's mother is reluctant to move house, as she has a good network of friends where she currently lives and there is no suitable housing, such as a bungalow, nearby.

The rooms in the house are all fairly small and John's mum is concerned regarding the lack of space for equipment. In the house, there is no dining area; the family tend to eat their dinner off trays on their knees, sitting on the couch in front of the television. The only seating in the living room is a couch and two soft, low armchairs.

At school, John is in a busy class of 30 children. The school is on two levels, although John's classroom is on the ground floor. The library and learning support base are upstairs.

There is a part-time classroom assistant in John's class and he has two teachers who job share. In the dining area, the children all sit on stools at fold-down tables. John is not particularly stable on this and the staff have been concerned for some time.

John's teachers have never had a child with physical disabilities in their class before and are becoming increasingly concerned about his mobility and safety.

## STUDY QUESTIONS

- What do you feel are the areas of potential difficulty?
- What factors would you need to take into consideration when exploring seating at home?
- What do you feel the solutions to John's seating needs at home might be?
- What issues do you feel would be important to address at school?
- How can the seating in the classroom be improved?
- What are your thoughts regarding John's seating within the dining room? Would you make any recommendations?
- How would you try to ensure that your recommendations were implemented and followed through?

# 7 Moving and Handling

KATE STONE AND CLAIRE TESTER

## INTRODUCTION

Occupational therapists involved in the manual handling of children, young people and adults have a responsibility to carry out a risk assessment for all moving and handling tasks. The risk assessment identifies all potential problems and is the basis for eliminating or reducing hazards for the people engaged in the task (College of Occupational Therapists, 2006a).

All risk assessments and manual handling practices should take into account the current legislation relating to the safety of people being handled and the person who is moving them. The College of Occupational Therapists (2006b) reports that the main pieces of legislation that have to be considered in manual handling are the following:

- Heath and Safety at Work Act 1974;
- Management of Health and Safety at Work Regulations 1999;
- Manual Handling Operations Regulations 1992.

It is important to be aware of the laws relating to moving and handling but it is equally vital that each person and their carers' wishes are taken into account when carrying out risk assessments. Under the Carers and Disabled Children Act 2000, carers have the right to an assessment of their own needs, which should consider their ability to carry out moving and handling tasks.

Other factors that have to be taken into account when carrying out risk assessments are the environment in which the moving is taking place, the equipment required for the task, the skill of the handler and the physical condition of the person being moved. Once the risk assessment is completed, all the findings should be recorded, giving details of the preventative and protective measures in place. It should also detail what further actions need to be taken to reduce risk (Dimond, 2004).

Moving and handling includes techniques for transferring safely, involving lifting, pushing, pulling or carrying. It is necessary to have up-to-date training in moving and handling and this is usually provided annually for health professionals. Training for parents is seldom provided and parents understandably create their own moving and handling techniques that are often unsafe.

People with Duchenne muscular dystrophy will need to be moved and handled as their physical abilities deteriorate. Occupational therapists need to be sensitive to the parents' and young man's attitude to manual handling to ensure that safe procedures are introduced at the correct time for the family (Silcox, 2003).

## WHEN DOES MOVING AND HANDLING NEED TO BE INTRODUCED?

It is helpful to provide parents of all young children with the following basic techniques to care for their backs:

- to stand with a secure base, with legs at hips' width;
- to maintain the natural curve of the spine without stress, namely not stooping to lift;
- to keep the load that one is carrying close.

These three core principles in moving and handling can be safely shared and can provide a parent with sound basic techniques.

A child can be introduced to basic moving and handling approaches early on in order to maximise the ability to manoeuvre with minimum assistance, such as for sitting up in bed or transferring into a car. This can involve small pieces of equipment such as a soft turning disc for sitting on for car transfers. In this way, moving and handling equipment can be introduced as a positive experience.

As the child's proximal muscles deteriorate, he will need increasingly more support. Regular risk assessments to determine the level of support needed must be carried out by a manual handler trained in moving and handling assessment procedures. An example of a risk-assessment guide has been included in Appendix V.

A boy with Duchenne muscular dystrophy is encouraged to be ambulant and mobile for as long as his skills and strength will allow. Moving and handling approaches must reflect this and enable him to be as independent as possible. The age at which a child begins to use a manual wheelchair varies, but it is often around 12 years of age. The time at which he will progress to a power chair depends on upper-body strength.

When a child or young person can no longer carry out a standing transfer safely, then he will need to be lifted. This requires a hoist. Manual hoists are large pieces of equipment and are often perceived as a tangible aspect of disability by the family according to Conneeley (1998). For this reason, a hoist might be initially refused by parents who would prefer to manually handle their son rather than use equipment to physically lift him. A coping strategy for many parents is to physically lift their son as his motor skills are lost. Parents have described this as originating from an action when the child was younger, often describing it as a way of hugging their son, and as an immediate and quick way of transferring their son. However, the number of transfers in a day can be significant: in the morning, from bed to wheelchair, from wheelchair to toilet, toilet to shower, to bed for dressing, from bed to chair, and from chair to car for school.

As the child grows bigger and heavier, it often requires both parents to lift and assist with manoeuvres. Considerations of dignity and privacy need to be considered. As the young man becomes older. It is not appropriate for a teenage boy to be carried by his mother to be put onto the toilet when pants and trousers have been pulled down.

For some boys with Duchenne muscular dystrophy, their body weight may be quite heavy. This does not necessarily reflect their diet or the amount they eat. In fact, some boys will try and limit their food intake in order not to gain weight and 'to make it easier for Mum and Dad to lift me', said one 12-year-old. This eating behaviour should not be encouraged, as it is detrimental to the boy. Boys with Duchenne muscular dystrophy have difficulties eating as they become weaker and slower. They often do not eat very well and sometimes require food supplements.

If a small manual hoist is introduced early to a child and family at school or in a hospice as part of the day-to-day caring, it can be accepted more easily. The overhead hoist is often the preferred option for the home but may not be installed until the child has reached his teens. Where possible, the young person should operate the remote control for the hoist and be actively involved in transfers as much as is possible.


## NEEDS OF THE INDIVIDUAL REQUIRING ASSISTANCE

When moving and handling approaches have to be introduced to a young person with Duchenne muscular dystrophy, account must be taken of his individual needs, wishes and cultural background (Heywood, 2001). His moving and handling needs and the needs of his family and carers will change over time; therefore, regular reviews need to be carried out. Before any handling task is carried out, it should be explained and consent given for the move. The highest level of privacy and dignity must be instituted for the person being moved. If there are communication or language problems, other ways of preparing and warning him that he is to be moved must be introduced.

Obviously, as a child gets older, they get longer and heavier. The techniques and equipment used to move a child of four will be quite different from those used to move a man of 24. Postural issues such as trunk and head control have to be assessed to ensure that any equipment or movement approaches used have the right level of support, such as chairs with lateral supports or slings with head supports.

The condition of the young person's skin will also influence moving and handling methods. If his skin is vulnerable, make sure that any equipment used will not cause soreness or rubbing. Carers also need to ensure that they are not wearing jewellery or belts, etc. that could dig into or rub his skin while he is being moved (Dare & O'Donovan, 2002). As the young man becomes less able to move himself in a chair, pressure will need to be relieved on the buttocks, even when there is a pressure cushion. This may require assisted movement from side to side or hoisting onto a bed. Where a person is in pain, moving and handling should be kept to an absolute minimum, except when it is used to relieve pain.

## INDIVIDUAL CAPABILITY OF THE HANDLER

It is the responsibility of all employers to ensure that employees are suitably trained to carry out moving and handling tasks (Mandelstam, 1999). They also have to ensure that the handler has the physical ability to carry out the number of moving and handling operations expected during a normal working day. Dimond (2004) advises that the employee and the employer have to make sure that the handler is wearing clothing suitable for the task.

In school and care settings, moving and handling guidelines are provided for the health and safety of clients and staff. Conflict can arise if parents who insist on carrying their son without the help of equipment expect carers to do the same at home or in other settings. Over time, parents may sustain injuries, which can become chronic conditions, such as back pain, shoulder and wrist injuries. Whilst staff have guidelines and legislation to support them in the safe moving and handling of others, parents in their own home can choose whether they use equipment or not. Accidents do occur, despite best intentions; one example is of a father tripping and falling whilst carrying his 12-year-old son. Conneeley (1998) advises that where there is a reluctance to accept lifting equipment, the members of the family may need more time to come to terms with the functional loss of abilities in the person with muscular dystrophy.

Occupational therapists (Stewart & Neyerlin-Beale, 2000) can provide advice regarding the number of transfers required and can also advise on how to eliminate unnecessary moves. Carers can benefit from advice on how to assess their own capabilities in moving and handling in the home. Such discussions can be helpful, as members of the family involved in moving and handling may have existing medical problems and they may require guidance in different techniques and approaches.

## ENVIRONMENTAL CONSIDERATIONS

The space available to carry out manual handling tasks can determine the method adopted. If space is very limited within the family home, it may be impossible to use a mobile hoist or to have two carers assisting with a move. If there is not enough space to carry out safe manoeuvres, this needs to be highlighted in the risk assessment, along with recommendations of how to change the situation. Lack of space can result in the handlers having to adopt unnatural postures, states Mandelstam (1999), which heightens the risk of injury to the handlers and the person being moved.

Furniture may have to be repositioned in a room to enable safe moving and handling procedures to be carried out. This can cause further disruption to a family and needs to be discussed sensitively. Floor surfaces need to be kept clear for all moving and handling manoeuvres. Particular care is needed where there are wet or uneven floor areas. The temperature of the environment should also be comfortable for the person and their carer.


## MOVING AND HANDLING EQUIPMENT

Occupational therapists are often involved in selecting and providing moving and handling equipment after consultation with the family and other agencies. Mandelstam (2001) suggests that where this is the case, it is their responsibility to ensure that the equipment is suitable for the task and that clear instructions are given on how to use and clean the equipment. This may need reviewing and follow-up, as equipment often needs to be demonstrated more than once. Carers should be actively involved in using hoists and other equipment during demonstrations.

All moving and handling equipment needs to be regularly checked and serviced. It is the responsibility of the owner of the equipment to make sure that the equipment is safe, according to the Provision and Use of Work Equipment Regulations 1998 (College of Occupational Therapists, 2006b). There is a vast amount of moving and handling equipment available. Pain et al. (2003) provide detailed guidance in their book on how to choose equipment for people with different physical needs. The following equipment list can help to reduce risk when carrying out moving and handling tasks.


### TURNTABLES, SLIDING SHEETS AND HANDLING BELTS

There are two basic turntables used to assist with moving and handling. One is positioned on the floor as an aid to turn a child who can still weight bear when transferring from chair to chair. The other is for sitting on and helps in getting into and out of a car or bed.

Sliding sheets are used to reposition people in bed or in a chair. They can also be used to help to position slings. There are a variety of different sliding sheets on the market.

Handling belts help carers to manoeuvre the person and reduce the need to hold onto clothes or limbs while transferring.

## WHEELCHAIRS

Boys with Duchenne muscular dystrophy will eventually need a wheelchair. During some stages of their illness, they will be able to use their wheelchairs independently; at other times, they will need assistance to get to different locations. The Muscular Dystrophy Campaign has published a comprehensive book on wheelchair guidelines for people with muscular dystrophy.

## BEDS

A height-adjustable profiling bed with a pressure mattress can reduce, or make easier, the number of manual handling tasks that a carer has to perform (Harpin et al., 2002). The height-adjustment facility allows the bed to be set at the right height for the carer, reducing back strain. It will also assist a child who is still able to stand to get out of bed. The ability to raise the back and knee supports in bed using the remote control gives the person independent control of his postural and pressure position. A pressure-relieving mattress on the bed can also reduce the number of times that the person with muscular dystrophy needs to be turned in bed.

## MOBILE SHOWER CHAIRS, SHOWER TROLLEYS AND LIFTING BATH SEATS

There are many commodes, shower chairs, shower trolleys and lifting bath seats on the market. Deciding on which one to use will depend on where it has to be used and how many functions you expect the equipment to perform. If a chair is to be used in the shower and over the toilet, it is better to have one mobile chair that will serve both purposes and take up less space. If the person needs postural support when sitting in their wheelchair, they will require postural support in shower, toilet and bath chairs. They will also need padding on this equipment if they need pressure cushions on their existing seating. Pain et al. (2003) give detailed guidance on selecting bathing equipment and highlight the factors to consider when choosing between a shower and a bath.

## HOISTS

A young man with Duchenne muscular dystrophy will probably use a variety of different hoists throughout his life, as it is unlikely that there will be the same hoist at every location. What is important is that the hoist provided will safely lift his weight and that there is no risk of him being injured by any part of the hoist and sling. This can happen if the boom of the hoist is too near his face or the wrong type of sling is used with the hoist.

The environment, the carer and the person with muscular dystrophy will generally determine what type of hoist and sling will be selected. Listening to what the people using the hoist want and giving them control in selecting equipment will enhance acceptance of the hoist (Conneeley, 1998). If the hoist has to be used in a number of different locations within one building or out-doors, a mobile hoist is better. If it only has to be used in one room, it is better to have a tracking hoist or a wall hoist, as they take up less space.

In the person's home, a tracking hoist is the preferred option, as it is less obtrusive and easier for carers to operate. Ideally, the tracking hoist should run from the bedroom to an adjacent bathroom to allow access to the toilet and bath. If the house is on more than one level, two hoists may be required.

## SLINGS

Depending on the hoist design, slings are made with loops, rings or clips to attach to the hoist. Some sling manufacturers will make slings with all of these attachment features, so that they can be used on any hoist. This is useful if different hoists are used. A number of companies now make specific slings for people with muscular dystrophy. Boys become familiar and comfortable with their own sling and occasionally can find it hard to change to another sling. Slings need to be replaced on a regular basis as the physical support needs of the boys change. Slings also wear out and should be regularly checked for faults.

Normally, a number of slings are used for different purposes. Mesh slings are used for bathing, as they dry quickly. When a sling has been used for toileting, bathing or against the bare skin of a person, it cannot be used for another individual until it is washed, due to the need to control infection. Non-slip slings should not get wet, as they cling to the skin. A toilet sling is not suitable for a boy with Duchenne muscular dystrophy, as full trunk control is required (Harpin, 2000). Toileting preferences differ and some young adults may prefer to sit in a sling over a bed pan. There are different commodes on the market incorporating shower seats, which can be explored; these enable sitting over a commode pan or toilet, rather than being suspended over it.

Padded slings should be used where the person's skin is vulnerable. These are more comfortable and will reduce the risk of the sling cutting into the thighs of the young person. Padded slings can take a while to dry, so check whether they can be tumble dried.

Slings should not be left in a chair or left under someone, as they can cause additional pressure areas and sweating, and can be slippery so a seating position can change. Slings can be easily placed and removed. If there is difficulty in positioning a sling, then it may be either the technique or the sling that needs changing. Most young men with Duchenne muscular dystrophy will need slings which provide head support by the time they reach their mid-teens.

## STAIRCLIMBERS AND LIFTS

Stairclimbers and lifts are obviously used to move people and so they can be deemed manual handling equipment. Stairclimbers are often operated by carers, who therefore need training in how to use each individual stairclimber. The company supplying the stairclimber should be asked to check that it is suitable for the person in the wheelchair being moved, the stairs and for the person who has to operate the stairclimber. If the carer is operating a stair lift or platform lift, they should also have training in how to operate the lift and how to transfer the person with muscular dystrophy on and off the lift.

## KEY POINTS

• Risk assessments should be completed for all moving and handling tasks.
• All employees should have regular moving and handling training.
• There are no standard solutions, as every individual's needs are different.
• Introduce moving and handling in a sensitive manner to the family.
• Ensure that all equipment is safe to use before carrying out any task.
• Ask the person whether they are ready to be moved.

## CASE STUDY

A young boy attends a special needs school. He uses a wheelchair for mobility. There are seven steps up to the house; these are communal stairs. The boy uses an internal stair lift within his home to access the bedroom and bathroom. His mother carries the boy up and down the external stairs to access transport and the school bus. She also lifts him off and on the stair lift. She now has a back injury and cannot lift her son. There are no other family members. The boy is due back from school. How can you, as an occupational therapist, ensure that the child could safely get to bed at the end of the day?

## STUDY QUESTIONS

• Who is responsible for servicing equipment?
• What type of sling is suitable for a person with Duchenne muscular dystrophy?

- What should a handler remove before carrying out moving and handling tasks?
- Why would carers or parents refuse to use a hoist?

## SOLUTION

The boy's mother could not have looked after any of the boy's physical needs, as she was in too much pain. The occupational therapist contacted the school that the boy attended as a day pupil; it was a residential school. The school agreed to provide emergency respite for the boy for a few days until a longer-term solution could be found. The boy and his mother were happy with this solution, as he would be spending time with his friends. Funding was sourced from the social work department to employ two people who were willing and able to lift the boy in and out of the house. Home care provided carers to help get the boy up and ready for school and to help get him to bed at night. The family agreed to look at alternative housing following this episode and were re-housed in a barrier-free home within a few months.

# 8 Occupational Therapy in Education

ALEX HOWARTH, HEATHER McANDREW,
MARY McCUTCHEON AND NICOLA TRAYNOR

## INTRODUCTION

Children and young adults with Duchenne muscular dystrophy will face many challenges throughout their school career. With careful management and advanced planning, a pupil with this condition can be supported in reaching their full potential within the context of the curriculum and the social environment of the school.

In this chapter, access to the curriculum and to the environment within the school will be the primary focus. Social and emotional issues have been covered in Chapter 3 and it has been assumed that transport to and from school has been addressed and auxiliary assistance provided. The intention is to provide guidelines for the reader to facilitate occupational therapy input in an education setting with children who have Duchenne muscular dystrophy.

Throughout a pupil's school career, there will be challenges that recur through each stage of education (nursery to further education) but, on the other hand, each stage also presents its own unique demands on the pupil. Whilst there is a general pattern of progression of Duchenne muscular dystrophy, this will vary between individuals, causing each child to require different strategies and supports at different times. Equally, each environment impacts differently upon the clinical reasoning process.

Based on the authors' knowledge and experience, we hope to provide a resource that facilitates a flexible and informed clinical approach to occupational therapy in an educational context for children with Duchenne muscular dystrophy.

### NURSERY DEMANDS

At nursery, a normally developing child will form peer relationships, develop motor skills and the capacity to attend, and learn educational concepts, such as numbers, letters, shapes, etc. (Meggitt, 2006; Sugarman, 2001). A child with Duchenne muscular dystrophy may have difficulty adapting to this environment of interaction and the need to share adult attention with several other children, particularly if he is used to being the principle focus of attention at home owing to his condition (Hendry & Kloep, 2002). In relation to educational concepts, learning difficulties may become apparent: they are often co-morbid with Duchenne muscular dystrophy (Harpin et al., 2002).

## PRIMARY-SCHOOL DEMANDS

On transition to primary school, a child needs to learn to negotiate moving around the school; to achieve greater independence in personal self-care and organisation; to focus on tasks, attend to instruction and remain seated for prescribed amounts of time; to meet structured educational demands; to mix with large groups of older children; and to be more self-reliant in terms of peer-group interaction. Acquisition of handwriting skills becomes an important focus so that equipment and strategies may need to be introduced (Amundson & Weil, 2001). Auxiliary assistance also needs to be established in such a way that the right level of support is provided (Jones, 2003).

## SECONDARY-SCHOOL DEMANDS

The transition from primary to secondary school will make many demands on the child physically, socially and emotionally (Shaffer, 2002). In primary school, pupils are generally contained within one classroom with one teacher. Secondary schools tend to have larger buildings, with greater pupil numbers. Pupils are usually expected to move from room to room at roughly hourly intervals. This imposes greater physical demands than before. Relationships have to be formed with several subject teachers and fellow pupils. Workloads increase and more mature, independent and responsible behaviours are expected (Shaffer, 2002). For the pupil with Duchenne muscular dystrophy, this is happening within a context of decreasing muscle power and increasing physical dependence and can severely affect social interaction, self-esteem and motivation. Sensitive management and constant communication between all involved are essential to ensure that a pupil with Duchenne muscular dystrophy fulfils potential in their educational environment (Jones, 2003).

## CLASSROOM CONSIDERATIONS

### EXPECTATIONS

Children in early stages of Duchenne muscular dystrophy may not look obviously different from their peers, so that the expectations placed upon them may be greater than their abilities. Conversely, children who have a significant physical disability (e.g. in the later stages of Duchenne muscular dystrophy) may have lower expectations placed upon them and therefore not fulfil their educational potential.

All children should be expected to undertake work at a level commensurate with their abilities. Varying degrees of cognitive impairment can be associated with Duchenne muscular dystrophy (Harpin et al., 2002; Anderson et al., 2002). In general, a child with Duchenne muscular dystrophy may tire more quickly than their peers because everything demands greater effort (Chambers, 2004). Reduced respiratory function (less common now because of recent developments in respiratory management, particularly non-invasive ventilation) may also result in a disturbed sleep pattern, waking up with a headache and feeling sluggish in the morning. This can be aggravated by medications prescribed to reduce the effects of cramps (Bushby et al., 2005; Eagle et al., 2002; Simonds, 2004). Timetabling of work may therefore need to be considered, with physically and cognitively demanding tasks presented when the child is most alert and receptive. It may also be helpful to build rest periods into the day.

## ENVIRONMENT

The environment should be adapted towards integrating the child as fully as possible.

Ensure that the child can enter and leave rooms with the minimum of assistance. Handrails may need to be considered if steps and/or ramps are in situ. Door furniture may need to be adjusted: the position and type of handles may need to be changed to allow the child to reach; and hinges may require slackening to allow the door to move more freely. Doors may need to be widened for wheelchair access or free passage of specialist equipment. The position and clearance required by an opening door may cause difficulties with access so that re-hanging or replacement with a sliding door may need to be considered. Consideration must be given to whether the doors are fire doors and whether adaptations are in line with fire regulations. Local fire safety officers should be consulted. In new-build schools, electronically operated doors with push pads or pressure mats should be considered.

## LAYOUT AND FURNITURE

Ensure that there is a clear path from the door to the desk and to any other important areas of the class, such as to the teacher, computer, fire exit, and storage area/bookshelf. The position of floor puzzles, mats, etc. will need to be considered in terms of whether they are a trip hazard. This will prevent any unnecessary fuss and attention being drawn to the child. Another important factor that needs consideration is clear access in corridors and cloakrooms. Crowds of children as well as coats, bags, shoes, etc. that have fallen on the floor can present risk both to children who are ambulant as well as those who are wheelchair-dependent. A chair will need to be positioned near any area in which the class sit on the floor, such as for story-time, if sit-to-stand transfers are problematic.

## FLOOR COVERINGS

Wheelchairs move more easily on vinyl non-slip flooring than carpet. If a tiled floor is already in situ, any broken tiles causing an uneven surface will need to be replaced. A recessed doormat is safer than a loose one.

## EQUIPMENT

### TABLES

Tables should allow clear access underneath. There is a range of height-adjustable tables available on the market. Those with a wheelchair and joy-stick cut-out will permit closer access to the table surface. Height-adjustable tables will also accommodate future growth.

Furthermore tables may need to be set higher than would be expected to prop and support upper limbs that are increasingly unable to move against gravity. Recessed areas cut into conventional desks can also prove useful in this respect, such as in science for static equipment that needs to be manipulated.

The child may prefer to use their wheelchair tray as a work area, but this may set them back physically from their peers. Give a choice to the child.

### PAPER/BOOK STAND

A paper/book stand can help to reduce clutter on the desk and help to meet postural requirements. It is generally important to reduce clutter so that the child can reach for things easily.

### SINKS

Sinks should ideally be height-adjustable to allow clear access underneath. The basin should also be shallow. Automatic taps are best, but if they are not an option, long-lever taps are easier to manipulate than cruciform ones.

### MOBILE ARM SUPPORTS

Mobile arm supports are useful for some children and can be secured to a wheelchair or a table. They act by eliminating gravity and thus provide a greater range of movement. Please refer to Chapter 5 for further details.

## ORGANISATION OF WORK/TASKS

If the child has shoulder girdle weakness, work and materials should be placed close to the child to enable them to reach. Generally, materials should be positioned no wider than shoulder width and no further than fingertip position when the elbows are by the child's side. Any further away will force the child to use forward or lateral flexion of the trunk. This is both tiring and difficult to correct to an upright midline position.

## WRITTEN WORK/GRAPHIC SKILLS

Handwriting is a major occupation of education (Amundson & Weil, 2001). Once handwriting is established, it is important to assess the following aspects of it:

- Speed of written work – can the child keep up? Does speed reduce with sustained effort? Are they limiting their ideas to accommodate their ability to record their work?
- Postural changes – as the child's posture deteriorates, their preferences for recording work may change: use of a scribe once use of a keyboard becomes too physically demanding, for example.
- Legibility of written work – is it legible? Does legibility deteriorate with sustained effort?
- Curricular demands – what writing demands are made of the child? These will change over time, particularly around the middle primary years. It will be necessary to project into the future and to monitor on an ongoing basis.
- Effects of writing – does the child experience fatigue and/or cramps in the hands?
- Child's preference – how does the child feel about using technology? Would they prefer to use a scribe?

Children with Duchenne muscular dystrophy may encounter problems with pencil skills on account of any of the following factors: reduced muscle strength; reduced range of movement; reduced grip strength; reduced stamina; and postural and coordination difficulties. Learning difficulties may also be present and these can further impact on graphic skills. Possible solutions include:

- pencils grips (various types), angled writing boards, resistance provided by both the writing implement and the paper, paper stands/'page-ups' may improve performance in early stages;
- reduction in the amount of writing required, such as by using worksheets on which the child fills in missing words/phrases;
- word-processing technology, including voice-activation programs;
- use of a scribe;

- more oral responses;
- timetabling to allow alternation of passive and active tasks throughout the day to limit fatigue, such as listening activity preceding written work.

Both word processing and use of a scribe require the child to develop specific skills; this process should be integrated into the child's timetable and considered in relation to available resources, namely staff support and assessment/ provision of appropriate equipment. Consideration should also be given to ensuring compatibility between assistive systems for written work at school and at home.

### Information and computer technology

Computer programs such as Kid-Pix can provide an alternative/supplementary means of developing graphic skills. To an extent, computer games can provide a level playing field for interaction with peers.

### Word processing

Word processing should be introduced at an early stage so that it is seen as complimentary to handwriting. It is important to note that persisting with/ insisting on handwriting will not prolong strength or range of motion. A variety of software is available to introduce key skills and keyboard familiarity. Standard methods of teaching keystrokes should be suitable for a child with Duchenne muscular dystrophy, although forearm support may be necessary due to increasing muscle weakness at the shoulder girdle.

### Keyboard alternatives

As power and active movement are lost from the shoulders and upper limbs, it becomes very difficult for the child to extend their arms to the top and edges of the keyboard. Trunk flexion is used to compensate, which is tiring and encourages poor postural positioning.
   Possible solutions include:

- on-screen keyboard with mouse;
- mouse alternatives, such as touch-pad mouse, joystick, trackball or finger-operated integral joystick;
- compact keyboard, such as a Cherry keyboard; these retain all the features of a standard keyboard but are smaller in scale;
- laptop, which can be taken home for homework and can also be taken to hospital if the child has frequent admissions; specification will depend on the educational demands upon the child and the child's individual needs, and the child may require help to set up the equipment.

Factors that will need consideration when choosing a laptop include:

- durability;
- weight and size;
- compatibility with software to support child's specific learning needs;
- size of screen;
- positioning, namely if it is to be used on a wheelchair tray, how can it be raised to the appropriate height?

Some word-prediction software can be accessed via a mouse or single switch, such as Co-Writer and Clicker. If switches are to be used, an assessment of type and position will be necessary.

Voice-recognition software is another option. This requires a high level of cognitive planning and skill to be used effectively and therefore may not be appropriate. The software requires regular calibration to accommodate changes in the voice of the user so can be very labour-intensive when a boy's voice is breaking or when breath support for speech is variable. Background noise may also interfere with the effectiveness of the software. Another factor to be taken into consideration is that a child may not be comfortable using this method in the classroom environment, as it is necessary to speak aloud. As technology advances, voice-recognition software may become a more practical and less complicated option.

# OTHER AREAS OF THE SCHOOL

## TOILET

Within nursery and primary schools, cubicles are often the norm and, in boys' toilets, there is often a row of urinals as well. In nursery and the early stages of primary school, the child is likely to use the standard toilet facilities and may need additional support in the form of handrails, footrests and supervision. Problems with toilet transfers may be reduced through use of a raised toilet seat. Later, a fully adapted disabled toilet will be required to meet the child's changing needs. Indeed, as the child grows and the condition progresses, he will become entirely dependent on assistance with toileting. It is important to be aware that it is not uncommon for children to reduce their fluid/food intake to avoid the whole process (Chambers, 2004; Muscular Dystrophy Association, 1998). Safe moving and handling become an issue as the child becomes non-weight-bearing. Adequate space to assist the child is therefore extremely important.

### Space considerations

It will be necessary to accommodate the following within the toilet:

- large powered wheelchair – adequate turning space required;
- two carers/assistants;
- changing plinth to enable clothing to be adjusted before and after hoisting onto the toilet; and to allow for additional cleaning. Support should be provided by wedges or pillows to prevent the child's legs from falling to the side. The changing table should be heigh-adjustable with an adjustable back rest to facilitate transfers into a sling and minimise moving and handling risks.
- hoist – portable or ceiling track – many varieties are available;
- wash–dry toilet (optional) – as the child grows and/or after spinal-fusion surgery, their posture may become incompatible with using these types of toilets. It is sometimes possible to use a supportive seat or frame over the toilet to address this problem;
- support options: grab rails/frame/commode/shower–toilet chair – many varieties are available; a padded seat may be required for comfort and pressure relief and the older child usually requires head and trunk support; seat depth will need to be considered to provide adequate support to the thighs; good foot support is also essential and a footrest may be required;
- storage for slings/toiletries/sliding sheet.

**Factors to consider**

- size of the child and future growth/posture changes;
- trunk support;
- head support;
- foot support;
- space available;
- privacy and dignity.

Please refer to the section on toileting in Chapter 5 for further information.

## DINING ROOM/CANTEEN

**Environment**

There should be an accessible route to and from the canteen table.

**Tables**

Tables must be of a height to allow access underneath, either for a supportive seat or for a wheelchair. It may be possible in some instances to use raisers on a conventional canteen table to increase the height without altering the appearance. The child may choose to use their wheelchair tray to eat from but, on the other hand, may experience feelings of isolation if not sitting at the table with friends.

## Eating

Adapted cutlery such as rocker knives may be helpful from an early stage to help with cutting up food. As shoulder girdle weakness progresses, the child will usually prop his elbows on the table, hold the fork loosely in the hand, spear the food and bring the head forwards onto the food. The table must be high enough to support this method. An upturned box or biscuit tin decorated to the child's taste can be used as a platform to raise the level of the plate and decrease the distance from fork to mouth. It may be difficult for some children to use conventional cutlery and crockery. Possible options include:

• lightweight cutlery with built-up handles, such as ultralite;
• fork with a cutting edge;
• rocker knife;
• cuffs with inserts for cutlery;
• bowl with a rim to contain the food when scooping;
• non-slip mats;
• mechanical eating aids – these require careful assessment before prescription;
• straw for drinks – if sucking becomes an effort, a straw with a valve to retain the fluid level within the straw may be helpful.

## Diet

An immobile child may gain weight very quickly. This is obviously detrimental to health and increases the physical strains on carers. It can be tempting to give extra treats to the child but this leads to weight gain. The child should be encouraged to make healthy choices.

Often, the child tends to select dry/finger foods in order to avoid the physical difficulties involved in cutting and reaching the mouth.

## Support

The child will require support to collect food and clear away. Opening packets and cartons can also present problems. As the condition deteriorates, the child will require physical assistance to eat and drink. A reduction in independence in eating and drinking is common following spinal-fusion surgery.

Dietician and general practitioner referral may be useful to address issues of weight gain and constipation, respectively.

## GYM/PHYSICAL EDUCATION

In the early primary years, a child may need supervision with changing. In the middle years, help may be needed. Once the child uses a wheelchair, it is best if he does not have to change for physical education. This may need to be negotiated with the school. In any event, loose, comfortable garments made of natural fibres should be chosen; jogging bottoms, T-shirts and sweatshirts are best, as they are easier to put on/take off. Care should be taken if shiny tracksuit trousers are worn, as these may slide against particular wheelchair bases. Some boys choose to wear lined trousers/joggers to eliminate the need for pants to be worn. It may be possible to adapt some items of clothing for ease of dressing and undressing.

In primary school, before the child starts to use a wheelchair, it is likely that for swimming, assistance will be needed both in the pool and for changing. A hoist to enter and exit the pool will be necessary as soon as difficulty with ascending/descending steps is experienced. If the child is wheelchair-dependent, a hoist, changing plinth and physical support will all be required to undertake the task. Extra time will also need to be allowed, as, otherwise, the child will miss much of the lesson.

## PLAYGROUND

Support during playtime will need to be considered. A bench in the playground allows a child who is still ambulant to rest without being isolated. Before the child becomes non-ambulant, wheelchair access and the quality of the playground surface will also need to be addressed.

## FIRE EVACUATION

A Fire Plan for children with Duchenne muscular dystrophy is necessary to ensure safe evacuation in every area of the school. This is drawn up through consultation with the Fire Safety Services and therapists may be involved in an advisory role.

## TRANSITION PLANNING

Transition planning is complex and demands consideration of every aspect of educational life.

## FACTORS TO CONSIDER IN NURSERY/SCHOOL TRANSITION

A multidisciplinary transition meeting should ideally take place in January of the year the child is due to start nursery/school to allow maximum time for any support needs to be put in place. A nursery/school visit will need to be carried out to look at access and to assess for equipment such as seating, rails and steps, and to liaise with nursery/school staff.

The nursery/school may look for information about education of staff/ peers and other advice relating to the condition. Liaison with the Family Care Officer and school doctor can be helpful in this context.

## TRANSITION FOR ADULT LIFE

Transition planning for adult life usually commences at the young person's Future Needs Review, which usually takes place in the third year of secondary school. Representatives from education, social work and occasionally the Careers Service will be present, together with the family and young person. The Social Work Department should be involved at this stage and should have carried out a Future Needs Assessment and/or a Community Care Assessment to determine the needs of the young person.

Even with the best of planning, there can be a great deal of change between the third and sixth year of school. There may be a change in the young person's health and physical well-being, family circumstances and educational goals, for example. For these reasons, ongoing monitoring is necessary, together with a flexible approach to service delivery.

Medical advances have led to a dramatic increase in life expectancy for those with Duchenne muscular dystrophy. As a consequence of this, professionals have to change their expectations of the young person with whom they work. Service providers at this time also have to adapt services to meet these altered expectations.

## FACTORS TO CONSIDER DURING TRANSITION

The occupational therapist, as part of the medical/social-care team, must plan to hand over the care of the young person to the appropriate adult services teams/professionals. This might include the community occupational therapist, adult neurologist and/or a physical disabilities team.

## WHERE DO INDIVIDUALS MOVE ONTO FROM SCHOOL?

Some will move onto further education establishments, to employment and to training programmes whilst others will remain at home.

Whether the young person chooses to pursue further education or employment, it will be important for the occupational therapist to carry out an access and support visit to whichever establishment is appropriate.

## ACCESS ISSUES

See Appendix VI for the 'School and College/Work Access Assessment'. This form provides a guide on the physical areas within the building to assess, including transport and fire evacuation. This will allow the occupational therapist to flag up any adaptations/modifications necessary.

## SUPPORT ISSUES

The young person will have a range of support needs that will need to be managed properly to ensure full access to work or education. Support workers will be necessary to provide assistance with personal care, such as toileting and meals. Practical support may also be required, to scribe, to photocopy notes and to organise work materials, for example. It will be necessary for the occupational therapist to liaise with the appropriate disability access officers within education, with social work staff and with employers with regard to the funding of the various supports that the young person requires. As benefits change and evolve over time, they will not be discussed here but it is important for the occupational therapist to remain informed as to those that are available to the young person.

## EQUIPMENT AND OTHER SUPPORTS

The young person may require equipment to support access to work/ education. Below is a list of items that may be needed. This is by no means exhaustive:

- computers with appropriate software – more than one may be required for carry-over at home;
- height-adjustable desk(s)/ergonomic work station(s);
- hands-free telephone;
- paper stand;
- advanced copies of lecture notes;
- hoist – several may be required if more than one building is to be used.

It is important to forward plan for transition due to the wide range of supports that need to be in place. This will ensure that the transition to adult services runs smoothly with minimum of stress to all concerned.

## KEY POINTS

- Challenges recur throughout each stage of education but each stage presents unique demands and each situation is different, despite the general pattern of progression of Duchenne muscular dystrophy.
- Normally developing children become increasingly independent during their school career – children with Duchenne muscular dystrophy become increasingly dependent.

- Clear access is necessary for both ambulant and non-ambulant children – all the various areas of the school, internal and external, need consideration.
- Timetabling should accommodate crowd avoidance, time-consuming personal-care tasks and energy conservation.
- Height-adjustable equipment can accommodate future growth and postural changes.
- Handwriting is an essential component of the educational process and takes up a large percentage of the school day; compensatory strategies and equipment need careful consideration for the child with Duchenne muscular dystrophy and constant monitoring is necessary in order to address each stage.
- Computer technology can play an important role in terms of both education and social interaction.
- Toilet facilities need to accommodate a changing table – toileting slings do not provide adequate support in the long term.
- Provision of equipment has to be considered, not only in relation to physical needs, but also in relation to psychological well-being and social interaction.
- Transition planning has to be carried out well in advance.

## CASE STUDY

Stuart is a seven-year-old boy with Duchenne muscular dystrophy. He has one older sister who is unaffected. The family lead a generally very active lifestyle and enjoys the outdoor life. Whilst supportive and caring, they are struggling to accept the implications of Stuart's diagnosis. Stuart has specific learning difficulties and frequently has episodes of challenging behaviour both at school and at home.

Stuart is beginning to find it difficult to walk for any distance and has become increasingly unsteady on his feet. Sit-to-stand transfers are becoming an effort. A manual wheelchair has been provided for use when necessary and the physiotherapist has discussed application for a powered wheelchair with the family. Adaptations to the home are also currently under way: an accessible ground-floor extension consisting of a bedroom adjoining a bathroom with a tracking hoist and specialist equipment.

The issue of forward planning for a suitable toilet facility at school, however, throws up several sensitive issues, both at home and at school. Stuart has developed a trusting relationship with his auxiliary at school and is currently accompanied to the disabled toilet but, once there, left to manage independently whilst she waits outside. The toilet is small and has a handrail to aid sit-to-stand transfers.

The occupational therapist has broached expansion of the current disabled toilet to accommodate a powered wheelchair and hoist transfers with school.

The current disabled toilet adjoins a cloakroom area on which several class-rooms converge. After initial discussion with the school, an application to the education authority was made, detailing the reasons behind the application. A copy of this application was sent to the headteacher. It seems, however, that the school is resistant to proposals to change the fabric of the building because of the loss of space and the disruption. It also becomes evident that they do not accept that it will be necessary. The next multidisciplinary meeting is quietly fraught for the occupational therapist as she tries to argue her case whilst remaining sensitive to the needs of Stuart and his parents in terms of acceptance of prognosis. No headway is being made with the school within this forum. Another factor that has to be taken into consideration is that Stu-art's auxiliary was leaving the next term.

## CASE STUDY QUESTIONS

• What can be done to persuade school to support the proposal for providing an adequate toilet facility in such a way as to maintain good working relations?
• How can the delicate issue of assistance with a new auxiliary during toileting be approached with Stuart?
• How can the laborious and time-consuming process of toileting using a hoist be reduced?

## SOLUTION

A meeting was arranged with the headteacher to discuss the school perspec-tive and the solutions that they were proposing. Support from a senior occu-pational therapy colleague was provided during this meeting and the Pupil Support Manager from the education department attended. The school's pro-posal for a possible site was discussed fully.

As Stuart very rarely opened his bowels in school, the school's first proposal was that Stuart would be fetched by his parents in the event of the need for a bowel movement or an 'accident'. The occupational therapists pointed out that apart from being highly detrimental to Stuart's dignity and self-esteem, this would not be an inclusive measure. Other issues discussed were con-tinence with boys with Duchenne muscular dystrophy; and the anxiety, disrup-tion and lack of privacy to both Stuart and his family.

The school's second proposal involved use of a toileting sling so that Stuart could be hoisted in the cloakroom prior to entering the current toilet: the toilet would therefore not need to be expanded to accommodate a changing table. Education had sought independent advice on the matter but the progressive nature of Duchenne muscular dystrophy had not been taken into account by the independent agent. The occupational therapists explained that a toileting sling would not provide sufficient support in the long term because of the progressive loss of muscle tone and postural stability. Although it had been covered in the application letter, the process of and need for hoist transfers and use of a changing table were again explained step by step. Stuart's dignity and self-esteem were also re-emphasised. The right to privacy was also raised. It was felt that the discussion could be much franker because, at this meeting, addressing the family's sensitivity in relation to prognosis was not an issue. Literature to support the application was also given to the headteacher and the need to start the adaptation process as soon as possible was reiterated.

With this degree of input, the school accepted the need to adapt the current disabled toilet at the expense of the adjoining cloakroom and a good working relationship was maintained. The toilet was adapted during the summer-holiday period so that the only disruption to school was reduction/relocation of cloakroom space.

The new auxiliary was gradually introduced to Stuart whilst his familiar auxiliary was still in post. A relationship between the new person and Stuart was begun on the basis of non-personal self-care tasks.

Stuart was introduced to the use of a urine bottle at home before beginning to bring it into school. For discretion, it was stored in a cupboard in the disabled toilet, to be taken home at night to be sterilised. Both home and the new auxiliary were trained in using it with Stuart so that the process was as efficient as possible and gave Stuart a sense of being handled with competency.

## STUDY QUESTIONS

- List the difficulties that a boy with Duchenne muscular dystrophy, who is beginning to lose independent mobility but still ambulant, would have using the dinner hall facilities.
- What are all the issues surrounding an occupational therapy recommendation for a major piece of equipment at school?
- Identify key factors in the transition from primary school to secondary school for a student with Duchenne muscular dystrophy.
- Consider that you are a teacher with a boy with Duchenne muscular dystrophy in your class. How would you explain any necessary equipment and adaptations to inquisitive classmates?
- A teacher is insisting that a primary-school boy with Duchenne muscular dystrophy is not making enough effort with handwriting, particularly when it comes to homework. How would you approach this? What would be the key indicators suggesting a need for compensatory strategies for written work?
- How could you facilitate integration in the playground?

# 9 Learning and Behaviour Difficulties

CLAIRE TESTER

## INTRODUCTION

Whilst Duchenne muscular dystrophy is a neuromuscular condition affecting the deterioration of muscle strength, proximal to distal, there may also be concerns regarding the cognitive abilities of the boy (Biggar, 2006) due to the lack of dystrophin, which can have an affect. It should be stressed that learning difficulties are not always associated with Duchenne muscular dystrophy, and that there are intelligent young men with Duchenne muscular dystrophy without any learning difficulties or impairment. However, as Duchenne muscular dystrophy is often perceived as the condition first, any other difficulties can be overlooked. Some of these difficulties are addressed here for the therapist to be aware of, and to address in therapy where necessary.

## DEVELOPMENTAL PROFILE

In the early years, the young child with Duchenne muscular dystrophy will appear slower to achieve his motor milestones, being slower to stand and to walk. This is 'normal' for boys with Duchenne muscular dystrophy. In addition, a child may present with delayed speech and language development (Biggar, 2006). Early intervention is helpful for the child and the parent in both assessment and therapeutic activities. These will involve the speech and language therapist and physiotherapist, as well as the occupational therapist in play activities. This delay in language may indicate associated learning problems and needs careful and full assessment.

A neuropsychological profile has been identified of boys with Duchenne muscular dystrophy as having difficulties in attention to complex verbal information (Hinton et al., 2000, 2007) regardless of the intelligence quotient (IQ). This is linked to short-term memory, presenting as practical difficulties in retaining information and comprehending (Hinton et al., 2000), and also affecting non-verbal skills such as carrying out requests (Bresolin et al., 1994). Also, there may be associated difficulties in productive language, not a dysphasia, which can be compounded by a difficulty in recognising speech patterns and sounds, too. This, in turn, can affect reading and writing. Such difficulties are to be regarded as a delay (Hinton & Cyrulnik, 2006) which can be improved with therapeutic input. The attentional–organisational skills also show improvement over time as the boy reaches his teens (Sollee et al., 1985; Cotton et al., 2005).

It is thought that the absence of dystrophin contributes to this selective cognitive processing (Hinton et al., 2000) and aberrant synaptic functioning (Anderson et al., 2002). However, there is progression with these difficulties as the boy reaches his teens. There are noted compensatory strengths of memory recall and visual perception skills (Hinton & Cyrulnik, 2006). There are other non-verbal areas of intelligence which need further research (Cotton et al., 2001).

## ATTENTION DEFICIT

Some boys with Duchenne muscular dystrophy may present with an attention deficit disorder (ADD) or Attention Deficit Hyperactivity Disorder (ADHD). These are linked to poor attention span, and can present as a range of behaviours which affect both learning and social activity.

The signs of ADD are given as: lack of attention to detail; inability to finish tasks; appears not to listen; failure to follow instructions through; disorganisation; difficulty in carrying out tasks requiring sustained effort; distractibility; forgetfulness; and loss of things. Separately, these signs are not indicative of ADD and may occur at different times for children under stress. However, if six or more of these signs persist for six months or more in different settings (Likierman & Muter, 2005), this may be an indication of ADD and requires assessment. ADHD is similar to ADD but includes a restlessness and physical activity, involving impulsive behaviour shown in speech as well as behaviour. ADHD can be more difficult to determine in boys with Duchenne muscular dystrophy because of the difficulty in physical movement. Behavioural signs are seen in social behaviour: interrupting others; restlessness; and fidgeting. When in powered wheelchairs, the boy will move quickly, and, at times, erratically.

The impact of these behaviours upon others is seen socially with the child appearing to barge in on games, of difficulty in turn taking and of difficulties in adhering to rules and order of games. This makes the child unpopular and can lead to his being excluded because of the behaviour rather than his physical disability. For some children, the behaviours may be perceived as an aspect of the personality of the child in terms of excitability, and are accepted by the family. But such behaviours at school can lead to unpopularity for the child in the playground, and trouble with the teacher if perceived as deliberately disruptive behaviour in class. Assessment is necessary, which may involve the occupational therapist and psychologist, as well as teaching staff. This is essential, as differential diagnosis can be made after a full assessment involving an interview with the parent, and observation of the child in different settings. As mentioned, emotional stress may be a factor for lack of concentration and restlessness. Also, any anxiety or depression needs to be considered with emotional-based learning difficulties that the child may have. Any bullying or social exclusion can exacerbate difficulties for the child.

The age and a history of the behaviour are part of the assessment. For example, many children starting school may present as restless and distractible as they learn the behaviour expected of them. In ADD, the child cannot change their behaviour without help. The child may show signs of frustration with themselves and others in trying to participate and undertake tasks.

Therapy interventions can involve strategies for coping for the child, as well as therapy. For some very restless children with ADHD, medication may be effective. Strategies can involve the provision of a simple routine and structure to the day, with tasks broken down into achievable short steps. The intention is to actively engage the child and to enable them to gain a sense of mastery, extending the child's attention span and developing their concentration span. Information can be provided verbally and backed up with written or pictorial prompts. The seating position in the class and reducing distractions is helpful to the child; e.g. sitting in a corner position at the front of the class rather than by the door or in the middle of the class is more helpful to the child. Intervention is helpful, for, without it, difficulties in managing the child's behaviour can occur in the family and with teaching staff, which can negatively affect relationships, social behaviour and the healthy emotional development of the boy.

## DYSPRAXIA

Boys with Duchenne muscular dystrophy may present as having specific learning difficulties associated with dyspraxia, which can be overlooked because they are not physically active and many assessments for dyspraxia are based on physical coordination and gross motor skills, including proprioception (see 'Resources'). Dyspraxia does not only affect motor coordination, balance and perceptuo-motor skills, but also sequential and consequential thinking, difficulties with abstract concepts such as time, and difficulties in 'reading' social behaviour and responding appropriately. Reading and writing difficulties are also seen.

Depending on the age at which the child is referred for assessment and the progression of the condition, certain assessments can be used. For example, these can include clinical observation of bilateral integration and right–left confusion. Avoidance of crossing the midline may be more difficult to assess, depending upon muscle strength and active range of movement. Assessment of eye movement is always possible.

Therapy will include strategies for school, and the focus on concrete rather than abstract tasks (Piaget, 1972). Social skills training can also be helpful for children (see 'Self-Esteem', below). Again, depending upon the physical abilities of the child, a degree of sensory integration therapy involving the whole body can be carried out. This has to be carefully assessed and constantly reviewed. Adaptation is possible with a wheelchair for some activities, such as slalom activity with cones. The therapist needs to reframe aims of therapy in light of the deterioration of muscle strength and motor skills.

## DYSLEXIA

Children with dyslexia may present with difficulties in sequencing seen in writing numbers or days of the week. There may also be confusion in direction of reading, both left to right and/or up and down. Letters and figures may be written the wrong way around, and this all affects reading and writing. The understanding of sounds and phonics can also be affected. Processing what is being read and written also takes longer for the child.

Dyslexia is usually identified at school when the child is involved in reading and writing daily. Dyslexia is not necessarily linked to a learning difficulty or a developmental delay, but does make school learning difficult for the child. An assessment by an educational psychologist is required and an action plan is made for the child. Useful screening tests are the Dyslexia Early Screening Test (Nicholson & Fawcett, 2004a) and the Dyslexia Screening Test (Nicholson & Fawcett, 2004b). Therapy may include the speech and language therapist and the occupational therapist in helping with handwriting. The use of a personal computer in class has been found to be helpful, especially when beginning secondary school and the amount of school work increases. It should be remembered that as the boy with Duchenne muscular dystrophy can tire easily, printed worksheets with questions to eliminate the need for the child to copy down work are helpful. There is no need to tire a child who has Duchenne muscular dystrophy unnecessarily.

Alpha to Omega is a phonics scheme recommended by the British Dyslexia Association (*www.bdadyslexia.org.uk*).

## BEHAVIOUR

Boys with Duchenne muscular dystrophy may present with difficult behaviours. These may be as a reaction to the restrictions of the condition itself and as a result of the frustrations and anger (see Chapter 3) or associated with a learning difficulty. Occasionally, boys with Duchenne muscular dystrophy may have a pervasive developmental disorder which includes autistic spectrum disorder and Asperger's syndrome, but this is not common. As mentioned earlier, there may be difficulties in social skills and in socialisation. Some may present as autistic tendencies, with a child actively withdrawing from the interaction and company of others (Mijovic et al., 2006). In addition, boys with Duchenne muscular dystrophy may experience overprotection from parents and do not have the same opportunities to engage in out-of-school activities, or even playing with local children and being able to spontaneously visit each others' houses. This contributes to a lack of experience and can foster an immaturity. For the child who also has a learning difficulty, playing appropriately with peers is more fraught when in a wheelchair.

As one teacher remarked of an 11-year-old boy with Duchenne muscular dystrophy who had a learning difficulty, 'He plays with some of the younger girls who push him round the playground playing "Mummies and Daddies" and he is the baby. He seems happy enough to be involved in the play as he doesn't have to do anything'.

Aggressive and angry behaviour may be linked to ADD, ADHD and dyspraxia, with the boys having difficulty in recognising social boundaries and acting impulsively. This should be balanced with the recognition of needing to channel aggression appropriately which occurs for all children when they become angry or frustrated. Usually, sports activities involving hitting or kicking a ball, such as hockey or football, are encouraged and this is harder to do for young men with energy and frustration who cannot participate fully in sports activities.

It is necessary to identify the impetus for the behaviour, the frequency of it and to engage the young man in ways of managing it. This does not entail squashing it and being denied the opportunity to vent his feelings, but recognising the need to channel this energy in the right way, and will depend upon the cognitive abilities of the boy and his level of insight into his own feelings and behaviour. This is important, as a grown man in a powered wheelchair who has not learnt to manage his behaviour can be very threatening as he attempts to drive into people and things. This is anti-social behaviour and, if encouraged through passivity of those around him, can create real problems for the young man and further isolate him. Creative ways of anger management which are appropriate and suitable for the individual need to be sought and encouraged by the whole family and with the educational establishment, too.

Oppositional behaviour (Mijovic et al., 2006) may appear as an attempt to gain control over the apparent overwhelming helplessness of the condition. Such behaviours can seem deliberately obstructive, displacing anger into those around them, such as refusing to speak or communicate, refusing to request the toilet resulting in self-soiling and causing real difficulties for the carers, or refusing food. Each of these behaviours is a form of aggression and anger, although they present as passive. The behaviour may be precipitated by a change or transition which has been difficult or even resisted by the individual. It is not enough to think that the boy or young man will give way or 'grow out of it' eventually, as some behaviours can develop and it becomes a battle of wills. Some parents may not be aware of any change in behaviour in their son, as it can occur outside of the home and be directed at teaching staff, carers or respite staff. Feedback and communication between parents and staff are necessary in such an instance. Individual members of staff may be made to feel inadequate as the boy refuses to engage or speak with them and, as such, staff can be reluctant to admit that they are having difficulties. However, any difficulties in a relationship need to be shared and discussed appropriately. As one member of staff said after several months of working with a young man with Duchenne muscular dystrophy who refused to speak to her in their one-to-one therapy sessions, 'I thought it was just me he didn't like'. For a young man to engage in such behaviour, there is an underlying problem which should be addressed with him, as avoidance and oppositional behaviour is a drastic attempt at gaining attention for their feelings, and it is the feelings and emotions which need to be recognised. Some basic strategies for parents are given in the Parent Project UK (PPUK) *Learning and Behaviour Toolkit for Duchenne Muscular Dystrophy* (2006).

## SOCIAL SKILLS AND SELF-ESTEEM

As discussed, there may be many different reasons for poor social skills. In addition, low self-esteem can result from a difficulty in socialisation and in reading social cues, but how are these skills encouraged and developed? First, it is necessary to ascertain what the difficulties are and the level of insight, intellectual and emotional intelligence of the young man, and views and atti-tudes of the family/teaching staff where any particular difficulties have arisen. This can provide an indication of difficulties. For example, swearing and abusive behaviour may take place at school only.

It is helpful to conduct initial social skills training on a one-to-one basis with someone whom the young man trusts and has a good relationship with. It is important that this is not a person in authority or with whom there is conflict. An agreed number of sessions in a quiet room which is easily accessed and private without interruption is necessary. Ideally, a fixed length of time (approximately 45 minutes to one hour) is sufficient. Regular dates and times are helpful and reinforce a consistency and sustained interest by the health professional in the young man. The occupational therapist may undertake the sessions directly or may act in a supervisory role with a colleague.

Before the sessions are set up, it is necessary to have a conversation with the individual concerned to ascertain his willingness to engage in social skills training sessions, which may be termed differently. An agreement needs to be reached on the date of the first session and where it can take place and the time. The first session is used to establish ground rules and a discussion of what will take place during the sessions. This may involve the drawing up of a plan for the set number of weeks (e.g. five weeks). The ground rules are agreed to by both parties. Confidentiality will be one of these rules. This provides an opportunity for the young man to discuss what is important to him, which can be incorporated into a shared goal for the sessions. A diary or log with these rules and the number of sessions together with the shared goal acts as a guide and prompt. All sessions should have a beginning, a middle and an end, both within each session time and across the sessions. The first session should be given to: the ground rules; the reason for the sessions; date and time, etc; and the shared goal, with suggestions of how this will be achieved. The last session is used for an evaluation and recapping of what has been achieved in the time. This may lead to a discussion of further sessions. The intervening sessions are used for the social skills training which will be specifically focused on the identified goal. This goal needs to be realistic. It may be related to anger management or a specific social skill, such as developing assertiveness and the difference from aggression, or speaking on the telephone, arranging to see a friend. Throughout the sessions, the individual should feel supported and develop confidence in his own abilities. 'Homework' outside the sessions may involve practising aspects related to the goal. Sometimes, role play can be utilised during the sessions. Often, the allocation of regular time and support of an adult who is genuinely interested in the young man is significant in itself and can effect shared understanding of the young man's difficulties and frustrations. Written prompts and simple strategies can act as a guide for the young man and a reference. It should be acknowledged that work through the sessions will not automatically change behaviour and also may identify who has the problem with the young man's behaviour. One example was given by a mother who complained that her teenage son had become argumentative with her and did not always do what he was told as he used to. This escalated to arguments which were not resolved. This particular 'difficulty' was linked to the parent not recognising the need for independence and choice by her son as he was growing. Sessional work involved both the parent and the young man.

## LAST WORD

Having inherited the condition of Duchenne muscular dystrophy does not mean that a person is exempt in some way from other conditions. For example, a person may have Down's syndrome *and* Duchenne muscular dystrophy, or he may develop cancer, or any other condition. It is always paramount to consider the person first and the condition second, being attentive to presenting difficulties and any new signs and symptoms which may be part of Duchenne muscular dystrophy or indicative of something else. Such assessment and

identification of developmental and behavioural difficulties need to be sensitively approached with parents, as the diagnosis of Duchenne muscular dystrophy of their son already affects them profoundly (Catlin & Hoskin, 2006).

## KEY POINTS

- A child with Duchenne muscular dystrophy may have an associated learning difficulty.
- Dyspraxia, dyslexia, ADD and associated learning difficulties and behaviours may be present.
- It is important to see the person first before the condition.
- It is necessary to consider the child as a whole in all activities and to identify any difficulties which may not be associated with Duchenne muscular dystrophy; the necessary support can then be provided.
- Other conditions and difficulties can occur for the child or young person apart from the primary diagnosis of Duchenne muscular dystrophy.

## CASE STUDY

David is at primary school, in his last year before moving to the secondary
school. His teacher has raised her concern at his behaviour in class at the start
of his last year at school. He is noisy and disruptive. She does not wish to send
him out of class but has difficulty managing him in the classroom. She raises
this concern with the new occupational therapist. The occupational therapist
discusses this with other teachers in this small school, who have all had the
same problem but considered it part of Duchenne muscular dystrophy. David
is having difficulty in reading and writing, maths concepts and in concentration. The occupational therapist meets David's parents, who explain that
David is having difficulties with his school work and homework, but they have
considered this to be a part of his Duchenne muscular dystrophy and to be
accepted. What might the occupational therapist need to consider and how
should s/he act?

## STUDY QUESTIONS

- What is the neuropsychological profile of someone with Duchenne muscular dystrophy?
- What learning difficulties might present?
- Why are learning difficulties not always addressed with a boy with Duchenne muscular dystrophy?
- Consider how an occupational therapist would approach an assessment of a learning difficulty.

# 10 Leisure and Play

KATE STONE

## INTRODUCTION

Like everyone else children and adults with Duchenne muscular dystrophy want to enjoy activities and visit interesting places, and their interests can be as diverse as the rest of society. Taking part in play and leisure activities can also be an opportunity to mix with their peer group or with people who have similar interests. Local libraries, apart from being a great source for books, music and internet access, often have a great deal of information on different activity clubs in the local area.

The importance of holidays for people affected by muscular dystrophy should not be overlooked. Lots of holidays are available in Britain and abroad. These can be holidays for the whole family or just for the person with muscular dystrophy. However before booking a holiday, it is vital to check what transport, support and accommodation the operator provides. Local and national voluntary groups have many holiday properties that are suitable for disabled people. Organisations other than travel agents and tourist boards can help to plan holidays and some will also help to fund holidays (Darnbrough & Kinrade, 1995).

Sport can be enjoyed as a participant or as a spectator; this can be at home or in sporting venues. There are many disability sports associations that can provide and develop sports opportunities for people with muscular dystrophy. Most sports venues, cinemas, theatres and museums are accessible and many offer reduced or free admission for carers. They also have a responsibility under the Disability Discrimination Act 1995 to provide information on what facilities and services they offer. Legally, offering disabled children and young people a less favourable service on the grounds of their impairment is unacceptable under this Act (Dimond, 2004).

Occupational therapists can assist families to source information on leisure pursuits, play activities and holidays. They may also be involved in finding funding and practical support, which helps each member of the family to share in their interests. Taking part in enjoyable leisure activities is a positive way to relieve stress and anxiety for all families affected by muscular dystrophy.

## PLAY

Play is a natural activity that is essential in the psychological development of children. It is a means by which children explore and master their environment. Development is dependent on the physical, emotional and social world in which the child lives, and it is important that a child with a chronic illness is afforded opportunities to play. Occupational therapists use play activities in treatment to enhance the developmental and functional skills of a child and to increase the child's enjoyment of play and playfulness (Case-Smith et al., 1996).

Noyes and Lewis (2005) report that children using long-term ventilation have to overcome even more obstacles to be able to play. They often have extended periods of hospitalisation that can leave them feeling isolated from their family and friends, and this can impact on their social and emotional development. Their ability to play may further be restricted by communication problems and transport issues. Long periods of hospitalisation can lead to withdrawal and a lack of playfulness in a child but, where play is encouraged, this normal activity can decrease stress in the child. Structured play can reduce anxiety in children admitted to hospital and it can be used to explain medical procedures in terms that a child can understand. Play can also be a valuable communication tool used by children to communicate their feelings and anxieties (Goldman, 1994).

A child with Duchenne muscular dystrophy has many barriers to overcome to be able to participate in play activities. Overprotection by parents and others can prevent a child from participating in play activities. Parents also need to ensure that children have enough time to play with other children, as they often have so many medical commitments that the time needed for play and leisure is sometimes lost (Muscular Dystrophy Association, 1998). They need the freedom to test their own abilities and limits in play situations (Dare & O'Donovan, 2002). All play activities should be based on the child's interests, not their medical condition. Activities requiring repetitive muscle-building types of exercise should be avoided, as they are likely to damage muscle tissue further (Harpin et al., 2002).

Where children lack the ability to position themselves for play and leisure activities, advice on positioning and postural support equipment can be provided to help the children participate (Anemaet & Moffa-Trotter, 2000). Toys and leisure activities can also be modified to allow access and avoid fatigue. This can be a bike with postural support, playing football in a wheelchair using a physio ball or using special brackets to fix cameras or fishing rods to a wheelchair.

# HOLIDAYS

Everyone needs the opportunity to get away on their own or with family and friends. It is still the case that most people with any kind of disability have to plan their holiday well in advance to ensure that it goes smoothly. Information to help plan a holiday is readily available on the internet and through travel agents. The Disabled Persons Transport Advisory Committee, Contact a Family and the Muscular Dystrophy Campaign websites all offer detailed advice on holidays.

## ACCOMMODATION AND TOURIST ATTRACTIONS

Most travel agents will be able to identify accommodation that is accessible to a wheelchair user but it is important to check what grade of access is provided. The wheelchair-accessible bedroom may be designed for a couple, with smaller rooms for children in the family. If this is the case, it could mean that the parents are left sharing a single bed. Establish what public areas in the hotel or holiday complex can be accessed. The holiday complex may be accessible but can the local attractions be reached by a wheelchair user? Find out what kind of transport is available to travel to different attractions and what facilities are available at the attractions.

## TRANSPORT ACCESS

Airlines have different policies, services and charges for people who are wheelchair users; it is vital to check what each airline offers before booking a seat. Check that the airports, aeroplanes and toilet areas used at each stage of the journey are accessible. Remember that aircrew are not allowed to assist with toileting (Disabled Living Foundation, 1994). Transferring onto the plane and transfers from the airport to the holiday accommodation need to be detailed to make sure that they meet the needs of all the people travelling in the party.

Most cruise ships can accommodate people with mobility problems but, as with airlines, check exactly what they can offer before booking. The ship may be accessible but some of the destination ports may not be.

If travelling by train, make sure that there is access to the train for a person in a wheelchair at the stations and that they can be accommodated on the train, as some larger wheelchairs do not fit inside standard trains. Assistance to get on and off the train still needs to be booked in advance. All new trains and buses should accommodate wheelchairs but it will still be some time before all public transport is accessible. When travelling, it is safer to have a head support fitted to the wheelchair, as it reduces the risk of whiplash injuries if there is a crash. There are concessionary fares available to people who receive high rate Disability Living Allowance and their escorts on British trains and buses. This allowance can also be used to help with the lease or purchase of a car for transport needs in Britain through the Motability scheme.

Most people, by the time they use a powered wheelchair, will need to travel in a car that has a ramp or a lift (Campbell et al., 2000). These need to be compatible with the wheelchair and the user. Always check that there is enough head height in the vehicle and that it can carry everyone who is travelling. When using a car, it is advisable to use a disabled parking badge, as this will enable you to park nearer your destination.

## TRAVEL INSURANCE

It is essential to check that travel insurance is adequate to cover all medical costs, including replacing medical equipment, when planning a holiday abroad. There are specialist insurance companies that will provide insurance for people with pre-existing medical conditions if their doctor states that it is safe for them to travel. It is advisable to take out comprehensive private insurance for visits to all countries, as a European Health Insurance Card only gives access to state-provided medical treatment in the European Economic Area and treatment will be on the same basis as an 'insured' person living in that country. This might not cover all the services provided free of charge from the National Heath Service in the UK.

## MEDICATION ON HOLIDAY

When taking medication abroad, it is advisable for a person with muscular dystrophy to take a doctor's letter explaining their medical condition and the medication they require. This can help with any questions at Customs or with medical assistance while on holiday. If oxygen is required while travelling or on holiday abroad, this needs to be arranged in advance with the airline and the medical services in the countries that are being visited.

## EQUIPMENT AND PERSONAL ASSISTANCE

If medical equipment or personnel assistance is required while on holiday, the person needs to decide whether it is feasible to take their own equipment and carer or they need to check whether it can be supplied at their destination. Special arrangements may need to be made for transporting a wheelchair and other equipment on the aircraft. If the holiday location includes nursing or personal-care services, they may already have all the equipment and facilities required, but make sure that all specific needs can be met.

## RESPITE CARE

Respite care can provide opportunities for the family or the person with Duchenne muscular dystrophy to experience new activities or to make new friends. There are many different forms of respite care, from overnight stays away from the family to holiday breaks for all the family. There are a number of agencies that provide and fund different types of respite care. Social services can provide information on these organisations and can advise on different ways of funding respite care and holidays (Dimond, 2004).

## FUNDING FOR SPECIAL WISH-GRANTING ACTIVITIES

There are a number of charitable organisations that will help with funding very special activities for children and young adults who are very ill. Each organisation has its own criteria for providing assistance. Website addresses for some of these organisations are listed at the end of the book.

# SPORTS

The number of sports and spectator sports that can give pleasure is vast. If a child with muscular dystrophy is interested in sports, introduce them to the sports of their choice as early as possible, to forge a relationship with the sport and others who are interested in the same sport. Active exercises and participation in sports activities should be encouraged to help delay the development of contractures (Bushby et al., 2005). Participation in sports gives opportunities to develop a competitive spirit, self-discipline and a way of making new social contacts, which can help to raise self-esteem and reduce social isolation (Chawla, 1994).

Sports can be enjoyed on many different levels. In football, there is the enjoyment of playing in a game or watching a football match on the television from the comfort of home to experiencing the atmosphere of watching a match in a stadium full of people. Supporting a team or following a sport of their choice can give hours of pleasure to people with muscular dystrophy.

Swimming can be good fun at any age and is an enjoyable form of exercise for people with muscular dystrophy. Check that the pool has a hoist to give access to the water and that the changing facilities will meet the needs of the person with muscular dystrophy. The building also has to be wheelchair accessible. Throughout Britain, there are swimming clubs for people with limited abilities where carers with special training are available to help.

Horse-riding for disabled people is available in many locations. A child in the early stages of muscular dystrophy will enjoy riding and it is a good exercise for helping them to maintain their balance reactions (Turner et al., 1996). In the later stages of their illness, they can still enjoy the riding experience in specially adapted horse carriages.

The array of other sports that can give enjoyment are too vast to list but they can range from wheelchair fishing to ice skating on purpose-built sledges. Most sporting associations will provide information and advice on what facilities are available.

## HOBBIES

The number of hobbies that people with muscular dystrophy can pursue is huge. When choosing a hobby, look for one with lots of graded activities that will offer opportunities to continue with some aspect of the hobby as the person's physical abilities deteriorate; in gardening, for example, the child could be planting flowers in the garden, the teenager could be propagating plants and the adult could be designing gardens for a living on the computer.

Collecting specialised items is another hobby that fosters social interaction. There is the experience of going to shops, auctions or special fairs to buy items such as special comics, games or antiques. Apart from the pleasure of owning the items, there is also the opportunity to exchange parts of the collection with others who share the same interests (Dare & O'Donovan, 2002).

Shopping, as well as having a functional purpose like buying food or clothes, can also be a social experience at the large shopping malls, where friends can meet to shop, enjoy a meal out and attend the cinema, music concerts or sporting venues that are often found within malls. With the advent of computers and the internet, almost anything can be purchased from home for those people who are not able to visit the shops.

The internet offers a lot of support and information to people with Duchenne muscular dystrophy and it can be a way of making new friends and enjoying hobbies, such as downloading music and games. When using the internet, caution is needed, as personal details should not be revealed (Harper, 2002). Computers can be used for many leisure activities and, with the advent of voice-recognition software and using environmental control systems operated by puff-and-suck mechanisms, this is an activity that can be carried out independently by people when they can no longer use conventional keyboards. The Golden Freeway Project (Souter et al., 2004) is a specific site for families affected by Duchenne muscular dystrophy. The original project was set up in the north of England and offered computers, training and internet access to families. Two objectives of the project were to reduce social isolation and to provide support to the families. Most of the 75 families found that using the computer and the internet enhanced their leisure time. Griffiths (2005) also states that the use of computers and video games in occupational therapy treatment programmes is beneficial to people with muscular dystrophy.

There are a number of interests that can be carried out with limited upper-limb function; these include reading and creative writing, painting, photography, graphic art and some crafts, such as model-making. These can be enjoyed at home or they could be studied at further-education colleges for leisure or vocational purposes.

Getting out of the house to enjoyable activities can be a treat that all the family can share. Days out to special gardens, museums and galleries, parks and zoos, to name a few options, have become easier as more venues become accessible and provide the facilities needed for all the family.

Joining organisations like the Scouts or activity-based clubs is an alternative way of meeting new social contacts or partners. These types of clubs can be an introduction to other leisure pursuits and can, as in the Scout movement, be a way for a boy with Duchenne muscular dystrophy to experience supervised holidays with his peer group away from the family.

People can enjoy leisure pursuits on their own, but Passmore and French (2003) found that social leisure activities were important, as they fostered feelings of self-worth and gave participants a sense of belonging.

## FRIENDS AND FAMILY

Friends and family are the most important factor to maintaining an active social life. However, it is important that the person affected by Duchenne muscular dystrophy never feels overprotected. They should always be encouraged to enlarge their social circle. Friends should be encouraged to visit them at home from an early age to help establish a pattern which will last throughout their friendship, as environmental barriers may prevent access to their friend's home in the future. Peer-group friends can provide opportunities for discussion about all topics, including sensitive issues that cannot be easily discussed within the family (Goldman, 1994). They can also help to keep their friend up to date with the outside world and their social circle when they are restricted to their home or are in hospital. Love and friendship from people can never be replaced, but pets with a loving and protective temperament can also give hours of enjoyment and company to people with Duchenne muscular dystrophy.

## KEY POINTS

- Play and leisure activities should be based on people's interests, not their medical condition.
- The Disability Discrimination Act 1995 specifies that offering disabled children and young people a less favourable service on the grounds of their impairment is unacceptable.
- Play is a natural activity for all children and children with muscular dystrophy need as much time for leisure pursuits as they do for education or medical commitments.

- The environment or the activity can be modified to allow participation.
- Check all the services and accommodation offered by holiday providers before booking.
- Check what funding is available for holidays and leisure activities.
- Choose leisure interests that have elements suited to different levels of ability.
- Encourage people with Duchenne muscular dystrophy to widen their social circle.

## CASE STUDY

The mother of a teenaged boy approached her local social service occupational therapist for help to fund a holiday for her son. The therapist established that the family had not been on holiday for a number of years and that the mother was not seeking respite care at home or hospice care. The boy attended a residential school in a different district. The mother, who was a lone parent, could not afford to pay for a holiday, as she was a full-time student. She was also a person who was very independent and rarely asked for help. The mother was also worried about how she could cope on holiday without all the equipment she needed to use at home to assist her son. Transport was also an issue.

Following discussions with the boy and his mother to find out the type of holiday they wanted, they specified the following criteria:

- the location was to be less than an hour's drive from the family home;
- they did not want to use public transport or fly;
- the accommodation was to be accessible to the boy and his mother;
- the accommodation had to be self-catering;
- the accommodation had to have a tracking hoist in the boy's bedroom;
- there had to be attractions near the accommodation that were accessible without transport;
- there had to be other teenagers to mix with;
- they could not afford much towards the cost of the holiday.

With the help of the social work information worker, the occupational therapist was able to identify a number of possibilities for the family and check that they were available for the dates that the family were requesting. One cottage that was suitable for a wheelchair user situated in a rural estate, which also housed a large caravan park with lots of entertainment and three different types of restaurants, interested the family. Although, on paper and in pictures, the accommodation seemed suitable to reassure the mother that it would meet their needs, a visit was organised for the mother to see the property and the surrounding attractions. A friend of the family volunteered to drive the mother to the cottage. The mother reported that the cottage would meet all their needs. The cottage was provisionally booked and a grant was obtained from social work services to pay for all the holiday. This included funding for a private tail-lift bus to take the family to and from their destination. The estate on which the cottage was located provided transport for the family to local attractions within a five-mile radius and offered free admission to all the caravan-park attractions. Mother and son both enjoyed the holiday.

## STUDY QUESTIONS

- Why is play important for children with Duchenne muscular dystrophy?
- Name three barriers to play for a child with muscular dystrophy.
- What obstacles could a person with Duchenne muscular dystrophy face when travelling by train?
- How can an occupational therapist assist people to participate in leisure and play activities?

# 11 Community Care

KATE STONE

## INTRODUCTION

Community-care services are crucial resources for individuals with Duchenne muscular dystrophy. Occupational therapists in local authorities can have a significant role in assisting people to access community-care services and therefore need to understand the legislative framework under which they are working.

The following pieces of legislation are the main Acts which direct the work of occupational therapists in social services:

- National Assistance Act 1948;
- Social Work (Scotland) Act 1968;
- Chronically Sick and Disabled Persons Act 1970;
- Chronically Sick and Disabled Persons (Scotland) Act 1972;
- Chronically Sick and Disabled Persons (Northern Ireland) Act 1978;
- Children Act 1989;
- NHS and Community Care Act 1990;
- Children (Scotland) Act 1995;
- Children (Northern Ireland) Order 1995;
- Carers (Recognition and Services) Act 1995;
- Community Care (Direct Payments) Act 1996;
- Community Care and Health (Scotland) Act 2002.

There are clearly many other pieces of legislation that impact on occupational therapist assessments and practice in social work, but the above Acts place a duty on local authority occupational therapists to assess and provide services (Dimond, 2004).

## COMMUNITY-CARE ASSESSMENTS

Occupational therapists working in social services have a duty under section 2 of the Chronically Sick and Disabled Persons Act 1970 to carry out assessments for disabled people, including children. The introduction of community-care legislation placed additional assessment responsibilities on these occupational therapists by requiring them to carry out community-care assessments or specialist occupational therapy assessments that can contribute to community-care assessments (Stalker et al., 1995).

Social work occupational therapists may also be asked to contribute to assessments carried out for disabled children under legislation introduced in the Children Acts and the Education (Additional Support for Learning) (Scotland) Act 2004 (Scottish Executive, 2005).

They may also have responsibility for assessing carers' needs under the Carers (Recognition and Services) Act 1995 and the Community Care Acts (Mandelstam, 1998).

Following the introduction of community-care legislation, many occupational therapists in local authorities were designated care managers. Care management is a process that starts with the referral of an individual for care services. If the individual appears to need services, an assessment is carried out and a care plan is prepared, detailing the services required to meet the individual's needs. Once the services are in place, the services and care plan should be regularly monitored and reviewed to make sure that the individual's needs are being met. The main objective of care management is to help people to live as normal a life as possible by giving them care or support that promotes independence and improves their and their carers' quality of life. It should also give them a greater say in how services should be provided to help them (Cooper & Vernon, 1996).

If the occupational therapist is the first person from social services to contact the person with Duchenne muscular dystrophy, they may be responsible for carrying out a community-care assessment. This is a statutory requirement under section 47 of the NHS and Community Care Act 1990. A community-care assessment has to be completed to ascertain the individual's needs and how their needs can be met (Clutton et al., 2006).

The purpose of the community-care assessment is to find out what kind of help and support the individual with Duchenne muscular dystrophy requires. The assessment must take into account the wishes of the individual and their carers, it should also encompass the cultural and religious requirements of the family.

There are different levels of assessment. Some are straightforward, simple assessments, such as those for a parking badge, while others are complex with many issues that have to be addressed.

During the assessment, the occupational therapist will have to negotiate its scope with the individual and their carers. The process of the assessment should be based on the expressed needs of the service user and their preferences. The occupational therapist will also have to establish the best place to carry out the assessment, as it is not always possible for a carer or an individual with muscular dystrophy to voice their opinions in front of family members or other professionals. During the assessment, the individual's and their carer's

expectations have to be clarified and they should be advised of possible outcomes and timescales for providing services. Guided by the individual's and
carer's views of the problems, the occupational therapist will then need to
establish the cause of the problems and try to reach a consensus on how to
solve them. The assessment should also prioritise the problems, taking into
account how the individual with muscular dystrophy rates them in importance.
The community-care assessment should also establish whether the individual
and their carers are eligible for community-care services. Finally, the assessment should be recorded and shared with the individual (Parker & Bradley,
2004).

Questions relating to the practical support provided or required for the
person with Duchenne muscular dystrophy and their carers will be asked
during the assessment. This will take into account the type of personal-care
assistance that the person with muscular dystrophy requires, who provides
this assistance and whether those assisting can continue to provide this
support. The family or carers will also be consulted regarding the support
that they need for them to be able to continue caring for the individual
with muscular dystrophy. It is possible that the family and existing carers
may not wish to continue providing care due to illness or a change in family
or financial circumstances. The occupational therapist may have to ask
other professionals or agencies such as NHS staff or housing officials to contribute to the assessment, as they may have important information that will
influence the kind of services that the person with Duchenne muscular dystrophy or their carer needs. They may also have to provide some of the
services needed or provide funding for services to be put in place (Davies,
2002).

Working in partnership with the person with muscular dystrophy and their
carers, the occupational therapist will establish the areas in which they need
help and draw up a plan of how their needs can be met. This is called a community-care plan.

## CARER'S ASSESSMENT

There is a duty on the occupational therapist to advise any carer providing
regular and substantial care to the person with Duchenne muscular dystrophy
that they are entitled to a separate assessment of their needs. The focus of the
carer's assessment should look at their needs, and not at what they are able
to do for the person with muscular dystrophy. The carer's assessment will
generally cover all areas of potential need within the carer's life. The assessment has to determine whether the carer wishes to continue caring for the
person. A separate care plan should be drawn up recording the carer's needs
(Silcox, 2003).

It is possible, following the completion of the assessment processes, that
there will be potential areas of conflict between the carer's needs and the

needs of the individual with muscular dystrophy. There may also be disagreements between the assessor, the carer and the person with muscular dystrophy, as each person's perception of the level of need and risk is different. When this occurs, further work needs to be done to try to negotiate a solution that is acceptable to all parties. This can occur when parents are reluctant to let young adults make choices, which they perceive as risk-taking, or where people with muscular dystrophy feel that their carers need a break from caring for them. If a consensus cannot be reached, then the different views should be recorded and the worker will have to specify the reasons why certain care decisions were reached (Heron, 1998).

SINGLE SHARED ASSESSMENT

The number of different assessments that have to be endured in order to get services often overwhelms people. In an effort to reduce the number of times that families have to repeat the same information to different professionals, single shared assessments have been introduced in some areas of Britain to encourage more joined-up working between agencies and to speed up the process for accessing services and funding sources. Written consent is required from the individual regarding which information recorded during the assessment is to be shared with other professionals or agencies (Cohen, 2003).

Assessment processes and tools may vary throughout the UK, but the same principles of assessment should be used when ascertaining the needs of any individual, be it a child or an adult. Good assessment principles are the key to developing and delivering the services that people need. Following the completion of the assessment process, the occupational therapist, the person with Duchenne muscular dystrophy and their carers have to work out a plan of how to meet the needs of the individual with muscular dystrophy.

## COMMUNITY-CARE PLANS

A community-care plan details the type of assistance that the individual needs. Once the needs are identified and prioritised, the occupational therapist, as care manager, will need to find out what resources are available that will meet the needs identified. These resources may be available from statutory, voluntary, private and community sources. In some cases, a friend or another member of the family may volunteer to assist the individual to take part  in some activities. There may be a number of agencies that can provide the services or help required. The individual and their carers should be involved in the decision-making process regarding service provision. When services have been identified, the care manager will need to establish who will fund the services. Alternatively, the individual or their family may request that direct payments are made in lieu of social-care services to allow them to have more control over how their care is delivered (Horner, 2003).

An individual with Duchenne muscular dystrophy is likely to have many complex needs that will require a lot of multidisciplinary working across a number of different agencies to meet their needs. The care manager has to have a clear understanding of each discipline's role and responsibilities and be aware of the services that they can provide for the individual and their carers.

There are occasions where particular needs cannot be met. The community-care plan should record any unmet needs and the reasons why they were not met. It is important to record unmet needs, as it provides evidence for developing new services (Dimond, 2004).

The completed care plan should have a summary of the identified needs and outline the levels of risk to the person with muscular dystrophy and their family or carers if needs are not met. It should also record whether the individual has agreed to what is proposed in the care plan and whether they have consented to the information in the care plan being disclosed to other relevant agencies.

According to Parker and Bradley (2004), the care plan should have a description of the level and frequency of assistance required and record who is responsible for providing each service. It should also note the objectives for providing the services. Details of what care informal carers are willing to contribute should also be recorded. If the individual or the family has to make any financial contributions towards the costs of the services, this should also be recorded in the care plan. Finally, arrangements for monitoring and reviewing the care package should be detailed.

## COMMUNITY-CARE SERVICES

The range of care services available varies across different local authorities, as do the criteria and resources for providing services. Resource constraints often mean that services have to be targeted at those most in need. A child or adult with Duchenne muscular dystrophy is likely to need a range of different services over the course of their illness. If an occupational therapist is acting as the care manager, they can help to organise community-care services other than those provided by occupational therapists.

Occupational therapists working in social services also have a role in providing services stipulated under the Children Acts and the Community Care Acts (Dimond, 2004). The main services in which occupational therapists will be involved are:

- assessment and provision of equipment;
- housing support and housing adaptations;

- specialist occupational therapy assessments and treatments to achieve maximum independence;
- support groups for individuals and carers;
- counselling.

The above services have already been detailed within this book, so this chapter will give brief details regarding occupational therapy services and will focus more on some of the other types of care services that may have to be organised by a care manager. These services are:

- home-care services;
- respite care;
- day care;
- help to take part in educational and recreational activities at home and outside;
- help with holidays;
- help with travel;
- care in a care home.

It is impossible to list every type of community services offered, as some services are tailor-made for individuals or local community issues.

## ASSESSMENT AND PROVISION OF EQUIPMENT

Occupational therapists are routinely involved in providing specialised equipment to help people with Duchenne muscular dystrophy or their carers to carry out everyday tasks. The range of equipment that can be supplied varies from family to family, but most will need the provision of hoists, postural seating, bathing and toilet equipment, along with equipment that will help them to participate in school and leisure activities (Pain et al., 2003).

## HOUSING SUPPORT AND HOUSING ADAPTATIONS

A core role for occupational therapists is recommending housing adaptations, which will provide better access and facilities for the families. The scope of these adaptations varies from a simple handrail to complex extensions that will provide wheelchair-accessible facilities. When adapting a house is not possible, the occupational therapist should support the family in seeking alternative housing that will meet their needs, whether this is public or private housing. Housing services have a vital role in providing community-care services, as they have responsibility for the housing stock. Though occupational therapists assess and recommend adaptations, they have to request funding from housing services for major adaptations to the home, as social-care budgets will normally only fund adaptations up to £1,000 (Clutton et al., 2006).

## SPECIALIST OCCUPATIONAL THERAPY ASSESSMENTS AND TREATMENTS

The occupational therapist can carry out a variety of different assessments, such as handwriting assessments, cognitive-functioning tests and mobility assessments. Following specialised assessments, the occupational therapist will often work with the individual to help them develop new skills or to find alternative ways for them to carry out activities.

## SUPPORT GROUPS FOR INDIVIDUALS AND CARERS

As well as providing advice and information about different support groups that could be of benefit to people affected by muscular dystrophy, many occupational therapists are involved in providing support groups or training sessions for families. These may be summer playgroups, carer support groups or sibling groups.

## COUNSELLING

This is an activity carried out by many professionals but occupational therapists who have developed close relationships with families are often involved in counselling sessions. This is not advice-giving. This is listening to the individual and helping them to express and explore their feelings with a view to finding a way forward with issues that are important to them (Bumphrey, 1995).

## HOME-CARE SERVICES

Home-care services offer practical help and support to people at home with essential daily tasks that they are unable to manage safely for themselves. This may be personal care, such as help to get into bed, or help to get washed, etc. They may also offer some domestic services, like meal provision, shopping and laundry.

Due to the level of care that people with Duchenne muscular dystrophy require, they tend to need large packages of care from a variety of home-care providers to meet their personal-care needs and their health needs. Individuals will also need help with domestic chores, leisure and educational activities.

Personal-care tasks at home could be provided by social work home-care services, private care agencies or personal assistants paid for by the Independent Living Fund. This is a national resource providing financial support to disabled people to enable them to live in the community. It can be used to purchase personal care from services or to employ their own personal-care assistants. Funding via the Independent Living Fund is only available for those over 16 who already receive social services support to the value of £200 per week (Kestenbaum, 1999).

Community-care services can also be purchased via the direct payments scheme. The Community Care (Direct Payments) Act 1996 gave local authorities the power to make cash payments instead of providing services for people with disabilities who are between the ages of 18 and 64. This enables individuals to have more control over their own lives. Subsequent legislation via the Regulation of Care (Scotland) Act 2001 extended the right to direct payments to children and young adults with disabilities in Scotland. In England, the Carers and Disabled Children Act 2000 was introduced to include carers, disabled young people and parents of disabled children; it is consolidated under the Health and Social Care Act 2001 (Dimond, 2004).

Individuals with Duchenne muscular dystrophy in the middle and later stages of their illness need considerable assistance to perform everyday tasks, so, when planning care, great attention needs to be taken to ensure that anyone paid to assist with caring tasks is allocated enough working time for the tasks to be completed to the satisfaction of the individual with muscular dystrophy or their carer. Home-care services can often have a dual purpose. As well as assisting individuals with care tasks, they can also provide respite for individuals and their carers, such as night-sitting services.

RESPITE CARE

Respite care gives carers a chance to have time away from the responsibilities of caring for an individual. Children and adults with Duchenne muscular dystrophy have complex care needs which need to be provided in a flexible and creative package. Ideally, any respite care offered should have positive benefits for the carer and the person who needs the care. A carer will feel happier about accepting respite if they know that the person whom they care for is going to have positive experiences while they are not caring for them. Parents spend a lot of time caring for their child who has muscular dystrophy. This carer role can suppress the parent–child relationship to the extent that it is advisable to offer respite care to the family so that parents can spend time together with them, participating in shared interests. This frees the parents from having to carry out personal-care tasks and ensures that they can have quality time together. Many parents do feel guilty about asking others to care for their child and they miss them when they are away from home, so it is important that the parent or main carer feels that they are welcome at the facility offering the respite. Similarly, some individuals with muscular dystrophy feel that they are being rejected when others are asked to look after them. Any non-emergency respite offered should be gradually introduced to the family until everyone involved feels comfortable with the respite arrangements. Changes to respite arrangements should also be introduced in stages, as even a change of staff or timing of respite can cause distress to the individual or the carers.

Respite care can be provided at home or away from home. Finding the type of respite care that meets the needs of the family can be a complicated task.

Each family have their own lifestyle and respite has to try and match in with this lifestyle. There can also be many different reasons for requesting respite services. It can be for a one-off special occasion or it could be for regular short breaks at set times to allow the carer to participate in other activities or to work. Sometimes, the carers just want a good night's sleep and would appreciate someone sitting with their child as little as once a week.

Some people find the provision of home-based respite an intrusion on their privacy; others prefer this option, as the individual is cared for in familiar surroundings. Another form of respite that is popular with families is the family-based respite with another family. Often, the families become good friends. There tends to be more flexibility in this type of provision for respite when there is a family emergency (Heron, 1998).

Others prefer respite in residential establishments. Here, it is important to check that the type of respite being offered will be positive and appropriate for the individual with muscular dystrophy. Respite can also be provided in hospices but the subject of care being provided for the individual in a hospice has to be very carefully introduced to the family and the individual.

The provision of respite-care services to individuals with Duchenne muscular dystrophy will have a constantly changing pattern throughout their lifetime. The most important aspect is to try to match the respite required to the needs of the individual and their carers.

DAY CARE

There are many forms of day care that may meet the needs of people with Duchenne muscular dystrophy. Arranging for the child to attend activity clubs with his friends is a more natural way of providing day care for the child. It can also be provided through summer play schemes and after-school clubs run by voluntary agencies. Day care for adults with muscular dystrophy who are not in employment or education can be more problematic due to the level of personal care that they require. However, with creative packages, day care can be provided for these individuals by using personal assistants to provide care for them while they are participating in indoor or outdoor activities of their choice (Dare & O'Donovan, 2002).

EDUCATIONAL AND RECREATIONAL ACTIVITIES AT HOME AND OUTSIDE

Restrictions on participation and inadequate access are the main barriers to recreational and educational activities outside the home. Parents are often more than willing to transport their children to activities, but, if they have work commitments, this might not be possible. Older children and adults with Duchenne muscular dystrophy may not want their parents to transport and accompany them to their social functions. They need their own space to develop new friends and relationships. Where this is the case, a personal assistant, who could be a friend or a student, could be funded to provide the personal care that the individual with muscular dystrophy needs while attending these activities. Funding can also be provided for transport and escorts to get to outside activities. The provision of equipment and adaptations also assists the person to participate in these tasks (Lacy & Ouvry, 1998).

## HELP WITH HOLIDAYS

Information is available to help people to plan holidays which will meet the needs of all the family. There are also many voluntary organisations that will fund and provide holidays for people with muscular dystrophy. Social work services can also help to fund holidays but grants for holidays are usually means tested. If the individual is not able to organise the details of the holiday, they can be helped with this task. Further details about holidays are provided in Chapter 10.

## HELP WITH TRAVEL

The reality is that people with Duchenne muscular dystrophy in the UK are very reliant on others for transport. This is mainly due to the lack of access on public transport and their need for others to drive them to their destinations. They will also normally require help to secure them and their wheelchairs in vehicles used to transport them. Details of who is responsible for funding different transport costs are available in Chapter 15.

## CARE IN A CARE HOME

If, for whatever reason, individuals with muscular dystrophy can no longer be cared for in their own home, residential accommodation will have to be sought. The same principles for matching respite care to the needs of the family also apply to finding permanent care homes. If the family and the individual are happy with the home and the care that they offer, this can help to make the transition to the care home much easier for the family during a very emotive time (Heron, 1998).

## IMPLEMENTING A CARE PLAN

Identifying and selecting the care services that can help the family is one step; the next step is to secure the funding to provide services. Many different agencies can be responsible for funding different services. The care manager needs to ensure that the services required can provide the care needed at the specified times for the individual with muscular dystrophy and that funding is available to pay for each service. If there are costs for services that the family have to pay, the care manager should complete a financial assessment to ensure that the family are receiving all their benefits entitlements. This process will make sure that any charges to the family are means tested. When the family know what the cost implications are, they will need to decide whether the care plan is implemented or revised (Davies, 2002).

## MONITORING AND REVIEWING

The more complex the care package, the more it will need to be monitored and reviewed to ensure that each service is providing a standard of care that is acceptable to the individual and their carers. The costs of the care package will also have to be reviewed at regular intervals, as the financial circumstances of the family can change, as can the cost of providing the services. Due to the nature of their illness, people with Duchenne muscular dystrophy are going to have changing needs as their illness progresses. Their need for community-care services has to be reviewed on a very regular basis to ensure that any extra input that they may need from existing services can be organised and funded as well as any additional services that they need. Service provision is not static, as agencies and people providing care change. When this happens, the care manager needs to check that the individual is happy with the quality of care that they are receiving and, if the response is negative, the care manger should raise the issue with the service provider to try to rectify the situation. If the effectiveness of the service does not improve, an alternative service provider should be sought.

A review should check whether the objectives set in the original care plan have been achieved to the satisfaction of the person with muscular dystrophy and their carers. It should also record any areas in which the objectives have not been met and comment on parts of the plan that have worked well for the family. Part of the review will encompass the cost-effectiveness of the plan – one transport provider may provide a better service at a cheaper rate, for instance. It should also reassess the needs of the individual and put in place a new plan that may require the removal of some services and the introduction of new services. Finally, a date should be set for the next review (Parker & Bradley, 2004).

## KEY POINTS

• The aim of care management is to enable people to remain living in their own home.
• Be aware of how legislation impacts on service provision.
• Good assessment is the key to providing good services.

- Care plans should be based on the individual's needs, not what services are available.
- Be creative when developing care packages.
- Community-care services can be provided and funded by many different agencies.
- The more complex the care package, the more it will need to be monitored and reviewed.
- Care management is a process of assessment, planning, implementation, monitoring and review.

## CASE STUDY

A young man of 18 with Duchenne muscular dystrophy requested a community-care assessment, as he would need support to take up his place at university. The care manager identified the following needs that would have to be addressed to enable him to go to university:

- assistance with all personal-care needs at home and at university;
- help with shopping;
- practical help within the home;
- transport to get to and from university;
- transport to get to leisure activities;
- specialised keyboard and workstation needed to use the computer at university;
- adult activities with friends after university and at weekends;
- a referral to community nursing services;
- extra support while parents were on holiday and on the days on which his mother worked.

The amount of support that this young man required was substantial and the times at which it was needed had to be flexible. The cost of providing the services required was well in access of £200 per week, so he was able to access funds from the Independent Living Fund. This was used to employ personal assistants whom he interviewed, who would assist him at home, at university and at leisure activities. The assistants were also insured to drive the young man's motability car, which solved his transport problems. His disabled student allowance covered the cost of a personal-care assistant at university, who also acted as his scribe and note-taker. In this case, a fellow student was employed for personal-care tasks at university. The disabled student allowance also contributed towards transport costs to university and funded a suitable computer and workstation for him to use at university. Suitable toilet facilities were already in place at the university.

Social work home-care services provided extra cover to get the young man up and ready for university on the days on which his mother worked and they also provided extra cover when his parents were on holiday. His elder single brother also agreed to stay in the family home while the parents were away from home.

## STUDY QUESTIONS

- Which pieces of legislation give carers the right to an assessment of their own needs?
- Name the essential elements of care management.
- What community-care services do occupational therapists provide?
- What is respite care?
- What is the role of housing services in community care?
- Why do care plans need to be monitored and reviewed?

# 12 Housing Issues

KATE STONE

## INITIAL CONTACT

The housing needs of a person with Duchenne muscular dystrophy are as diverse as the individuals. Many factors have to be taken into account before an occupational therapist can make any recommendations regarding housing for the person and their family (Bull, 1998). Occupational therapists have a body of knowledge regarding housing adaptations and can offer constructive advice on housing issues.

A house is more than a building – it is a home, and each family will value and view their home in their own way. These values have to be taken into account in all housing assessments (Hawkins & Stewart, 2002).

Initially, it is essential to establish a relationship with the family to ascertain what issues are of concern to each member of the family (Office of the Deputy Prime Minister, 2004). The stage that each member of the family is at in understanding and accepting the prognosis of the person with Duchenne muscular dystrophy needs to be considered (Emery, 2000) before any actions are suggested. It is vital to establish what parents have told the child about his condition and what they want discussed in the presence of a child (Dare & O'Donovan, 2002). The older child who desires his own privacy within the family home and the younger adult with Duchenne muscular dystrophy who wants to leave home must be heard.

Picking and Pain (2003) suggest if housing issues are raised, the problems should be identified and the occupational therapist should clarify their role with the family in resolving the problem. They may only wish to be supplied with the relevant information they need to help them make their own decisions or they may want the occupational therapist to act as an intermediary on their behalf with housing organisations.

On the initial visit to the house, it may be apparent to the occupational therapist that the house will not meet the needs of the family in the future. If the family does not mention housing issues, the occupational therapist will have to determine when the family is ready to make changes (Turner et al., 2002). Even if the family has not raised specific housing issues, a visit to the family home can supply a lot of basic information regarding their housing situation, which the therapist can use to help plan future actions.

## LEGISLATION

There are many pieces of legislation that can assist people with housing issues. The following are some of the Acts that can be used to help obtain suitable housing for people with Duchenne muscular dystrophy:

* National Health Service and Community Care Act 1990;
* Carers (Recognition and Services) Act 1995;
* Carers and Disabled Children Act 2000;
* Chronically Sick and Disabled Person Act 1970;
* Children Act 1989;
* The Children (Scotland) Act 1995;
* Disability Discrimination Act 1995;
* Housing Grants, Construction and Regeneration Act 1996: Mandatory Disabled Facility Grant;
* Community Care (Delayed Discharges etc.) Act 2003;
* Human Rights Act 1998;
* Housing (Scotland) Act 1987.

Under community-care legislation, an occupational therapist in social services may also have a care manager's role in which they have to assess and coordinate care services, equipment and home adaptations. All social-care services must be assessed for and provided under specific legislation.

A good working knowledge of the above Acts will help to establish who is responsible for assessment, funding and provision regarding housing problems (Clutton et al., 2006; Scottish Homes, 1999a; Office of the Deputy Prime Minister, 2004).

## THE EXISTING HOUSE

When checking the suitability of any house, the topography of the local area needs to be studied. The house could be situated at the top of a hill in a rural area or in the middle of a pedestrian area, with no direct access to the street. Look at the facilities near the house, such as schools, shops and transport. Some family members may have to use public transport. Is there an adequate service? Identify the family's support network and their location. This may be a major factor when considering moving house. Think about the distance that the family have to travel to employment and schools from their present home and from any proposed new home (Bull, 1998).

## EXTERNAL ACCESS TO THE HOUSE

The family will need transport and access to transport. Does their present home have parking adjacent to the house and is the parking area sufficient to allow transfers from the car to a wheelchair beside or behind the car? If there is parking, can the person in a wheelchair access the house from the parking area? Look for steps or paths that are less than 900 mm wide that would block access. Consideration also has to be given to the surface of the paths, as gravel or slippery surfaces are not suitable for wheelchairs or people unsteady on their feet. While viewing the area around the house, find out whether there is access to a garden area for a wheelchair user (Silcox, 2003). It is important that children with muscular dystrophy have access to the garden, as this will help with their development (Heywood, 2001).

When the area around the house has been checked, the next stage is to inspect the entry into the house. The external doors need to be 900–1,000 mm wide, to allow for powered-wheelchair access in the future. Check the number of steps at each entrance, as this may be a factor when providing a ramp at their existing house. How deep are the existing steps and do they have a handrail to give assistance to those children who are still mobile but unsteady? If there are too many steps to allow the construction of a ramp with a safe gradient of 1 : 15, is there an alternative area where a ramp, stair lift, porch lift or the platform lift that converts into a set of steps, for others to use, could be installed without blocking access for others (Clutton et al., 2006)?

## HALL AND STAIRS

Inside the house, the hall needs to be 900–1,500 mm wide, to allow a powered wheelchair user to manoeuvre. Check for tight turns in the hall that would block free use of a wheelchair. Look at heaters or other objects that would be a barrier to a wheelchair user, especially door thresholds and flooring. All the interior doors in the house need to be 850–900 mm wide, to allow wheelchair access; remember that most bathroom doors in houses tend to be narrower than other doors. Most powered wheelchairs need a turning circle of 1,700 mm, but this may not be achievable in hallways and bathrooms.

If the house has more than one floor, the sizes in the hall upstairs also need to be checked if the person with muscular dystrophy uses this area. Think about how the unsteady child gets upstairs safely. Are there adequate handrails or would they be safer using a lift? Check the stairs to see whether there is adequate space to install a stair lift or platform lift over all the stairs without blocking any doors. If the person has to be hoisted on and off the lift, make sure that there is enough space and track at the top and bottom of the stair lift to allow transfers using a hoist. Where a stair lift cannot be installed or is unsuitable for the person, look for areas within the hall or the house where a vertical lift can be installed. The lift needs to accommodate a powered wheelchair without removing vital family living space (Pain et al., 2003). There may already be a lift within the family home. Ensure the person with Duchenne muscular dystrophy can safely access and control the lift. If the person is at risk using the lift, recommend changes that will meet the person's needs or give advice on alternatives.

Storage for equipment is a major problem. Does the hall have enough storage areas and are there sufficient sockets for charging equipment? If there is no storage in the hall, is there space in the garage or an extra bedroom where equipment can be stored?

In all rooms, the sockets, light switches, doors and door handles should be accessible. Think about automatic door openers for people who cannot manage door handles. The doors should be positioned to give maximum access to the rooms. If this is not the case, think about installing sliding doors or turning the hinges on the doors around. Where this is not sufficient to allow entry, widen existing doors or create a new door. Kick plates are also a sensible addition to protect doors from wheelchair damage (Harpin, 2000).

All floors in the house have to be examined for hazards, such as raised thresholds, loose carpets or tiles. The texture of the flooring may also be an impediment to wheelchair users or to a child with balance problems.

## KITCHEN

Determine who needs to use the facilities within the kitchen. It may be the carer who is the main user. If this is the case, the kitchen utilities need to be positioned for their convenience. If there is to be dual use of the kitchen, provide a height-adjustable workspace area for a wheelchair user, where they can access storage areas and utilities. Examine the existing utilities, such as the cooker and the sink, and check whether a person in a wheelchair can access the taps and controls. These can also be height-adjustable with clearance under the sink and hob for wheelchair access. All height-adjustable units should be operated by electric touch controls. Check the circulation space in the kitchen (Skelt, 1993).

There are many pieces of lightweight kitchen equipment that can make it easier for a person with muscular dystrophy to continue using the kitchen. In the early stages of their illness, it may be enough to introduce energy-saving techniques, such as providing a chair or perching stool in the kitchen for them to rest on while they are carrying out kitchen activities (Harpin et al., 2002).

When major alterations are needed to make the kitchen suitable for a wheelchair user, confirm whether there is enough space in the existing kitchen for the adaptations. If there is not enough space in the kitchen, is there another area that would be suitable to convert to a kitchen?

## BATHROOM

The bathroom causes the most problems for people with Duchenne muscular dystrophy. One of the first things to check is the flooring. A child who is unsteady on his feet needs non-slip flooring. Initially, a child will need grab rails to assist with mobility and transfers. Is there space to install grab rails in the areas in which they are required? The walls also have to be checked to make sure they can support grab rails. There are a number of toilet frames and specialised toilets that can assist a child to stand from sitting on the toilet. These can also provide postural support on the toilet for people who cannot stand.

The variety of bathing and showering equipment available is vast. They range from the simple bath seat and bath board to hydraulic bath seats and wheeled shower seats. Pain et al. (2003) provided detailed guidance on how to choose equipment and assistive devices.

Examine the bathroom to see whether there is enough room to allow wheelchair access with sufficient space to allow assisted bathing, shower and toilet transfers. Would there be enough room for a mobile hoist in the bathroom? If not, could a tracking or wall hoist be installed? If a changing bench or a shower trolley is required, is there space to accommodate these items and allow wheelchair access? The fixtures in the bathroom need to meet the needs of the person with Duchenne muscular dystrophy and the family if there is only one bathroom. Consider the toilet height for transfers. Can the person with muscular dystrophy flush the toilet and dry himself? A toilet that washes and dries the user may have to be installed. If the person has to use a toilet aid or wheeled commode chair, make sure that it is compatible with the toilet.

Ensure there is access to the washbasin for the person in a wheelchair and ascertain whether they can operate the taps. There are a number of height-adjustable washbasins available on the market that offer a variety of ways of operating the taps for those who cannot use ordinary taps. Worktops beside the basin can offer additional support for people who have problems holding their arms up (Harpin, 2000). Taps can also be thermostatically controlled to prevent scalding and can also have a flow control to prevent flooding. For those that are still mobile but unsteady on their feet, check whether there is enough space for a perching stool to be placed at the washbasin to give them postural support while using the basin. Wall-mounted body dryers are also available for people who are not able to dry themselves but can shower or bathe independently.

The shape and height of a bath can determine whether bath aids can be used to help with transfers and postural support. Some baths come with integrated hydraulic seats that can lift or lower a person into the bath; they also provide an element of postural support in the bath. Some of these baths are also height-adjustable. If a mobile hoist needs to be used to access the bath, is there space for the hoist underneath the bath? If not, is there room for a wall-mounted or tracking hoist? When a tracking hoist or wall-mounted hoist is being considered, a survey will have to be done to ensure that the wall or ceiling joists will support the hoist. When a hoist is being installed, try and ensure that it gives access to the toilet, bath, shower and chair.

Where there is a shower, the controls should be accessible and thermostatically controlled. The shower head should be height-adjustable and detachable. What type of shower facility is present? Is it a cubicle shower, an over-bath shower, a level-deck shower or a wet area? In a wet area, the floor of the bathroom is sealed and there is a drain in the floor. A cubicle shower may have a step up into the shower or it may have a level access. The size of the shower base also has to be measured to make sure that it will accommodate any equipment needed to ensure safety while showering. The base has to be strong enough to support the equipment. When doors are present, does this prove a barrier to accessing the shower cubicle? Where a wheeled shower chair is to be used for showering, there should be a level access shower base or a wet area. If the person is to be showered on a showering bench or trolley, the hose on the shower should be long enough to reach the whole length of the bench. Showering benches – wall-mounted or mobile – should be height-adjustable to assist with transfers (Pain et al., 2003).

It is possible, in some bathrooms, to remove the bath and convert the space into a wet area, but this has to be carefully considered, as a wet floor area could be a hazard to other users. Before embarking on this type of conversion, careful measurements have to be made to ensure that the area will be big enough to house everything that needs to be used in the wet area. If the bathroom is not big enough, identify whether there is another area that can be converted into a suitable bathroom for the person with Duchenne muscular dystrophy. This also applies if the person cannot access the existing bathroom in the house. When adapting or creating a bathroom, ensure that there is adequate heating and consider how the finished bathroom will look. A facility that looks institutional, Oldman and Beresford (1998) state, is likely to cause great distress to the family.

## BEDROOMS

Establish where the bedrooms are located and how many bedrooms there are in the house. Check there are enough bedrooms for the family and for any carers who have to sleep at the family home. Is the person with muscular dystrophy isolated from the rest of the family and can the house be altered to prevent this isolation? Heywood (2001) stresses that this is an issue that also has to be considered when planning adaptations. Some parents are not happy to leave a young child alone in a bedroom downstairs when the rest of the family is upstairs. The child may also feel left out. A system for obtaining assistance that is accessible needs to be installed in the bedroom. This can be as simple as a baby monitor for younger children but a more sophisticated system needs to be installed for young adults to allow privacy.

People with muscular dystrophy need a bedroom in which there is enough circulation space for a wheelchair when all their furniture and equipment are in place. In all rooms, sockets and light switches should be accessible but it is of particular importance that they are accessible from the bed in the bedroom. The type of bed needed varies, depending on the progress of the disease. At first, an ordinary bed that allows clearance under the bed to fit equipment is all that is necessary. Later, the person may need a bed that allows them to change their position in bed independently or they may need a height-adjustable bed to assist with transfers or to help their carer (Harpin et al., 2002).

There needs to be enough space for a hoist in the bedroom, whether it is a mobile hoist or a tracking hoist. If there is an en-suite bathroom, check whether the hoist can be used in both the bedroom and the en-suite. A lot of time can be spent in the bedroom; therefore, there should be enough space for a comfortable postural support chair and a suitable worktop area. The person with Duchenne muscular dystrophy must to be able to control their environment while they are in their bedroom. They need controls to operate the heating and windows independently. If a great deal of time is spent in the bedroom, consider the view that the person is looking at from their bed. If the existing bedroom cannot be made suitable for the person, is there a better room available?

## LIVING AREAS

The reception rooms in the house need to have enough circulation space for a wheelchair user once all the furniture is in place. Check the flooring, sockets and light switches for access. Environmental controls may also be necessary in living areas to control the heat and light in the room as well as other electrical devices. Harmer and Bakheit (1999) report that the provision of an environmental control system can enhance feelings of self-worth in people who use them. They also allow them control over their surroundings and can help with home security as well as provide alternative ways of communicating.

## FIRE SAFETY

Investigate what provisions have been made for the person with Duchenne muscular dystrophy in the event of a fire, especially if they are isolated from the rest of the family at night. Identify the location of smoke alarms and establish whether the person with muscular dystrophy can leave the house independently.

EXTENSIONS

While examining the house, it may be evident that there is not enough suitable space to provide the facilities that the family need. If this is the case, consider whether it is possible to extend the house. It is a good idea to mark out the size of any adaptation or extension to ensure that the family knows how much space would be lost (Scottish Homes, 1999a).

## HOUSING OPTIONS

Following a detailed assessment of the family's housing needs, the occupational therapist can make recommendations regarding the suitability of the family's existing home (Clutton et al., 2006). The three most common outcomes following an assessment are:

- the family decides to stay in their existing house, with no alterations;
- the family stays in their existing home, with alterations;
- the family moves to a new home.

### THE HOUSE WITH NO ALTERATIONS

In exceptional circumstances, some families will have a home that will meet the needs of the whole family without any adaptations. They are, however, likely to need equipment to assist with the care of the person with muscular dystrophy.

Other families, Heywood (2001) states, will delay addressing housing issues for personal or financial reasons. Some families refuse alterations to the house, as they fear it will hinder their chances of being offered a new house or will cause problems when they want to sell their house.

### ALTERING THE EXISTING HOUSE

Initially, the family may seek help with very minor alterations at home, such as a grab rail at the toilet. These requests should be dealt with at a pace that all the family can cope with, as offering too much assistance or too little assistance can jeopardise the occupational therapist's relationship with the family. Care also has to be taken to ensure that a child is not pushed too early into a dependent role by the provision of equipment.

When the family get to a point at which they are considering major adaptations to their property, they need to have good advice about the different alternatives available to enable them to make an informed choice before proceeding. The Muscular Dystrophy Campaign has produced an excellent adaptations manual by Harpin (2000) that guides you through the procedures.

Ideally, the family should be able to view a similar adaptation to ensure that it is really what they have envisioned. They should also be aware of how much space the adaptation will need, such as how much of their garden they will lose if a ramp or extension is constructed. The time needed for the adaptation from planning to completion should be explained to the family, as many will not realise how long the process may take (Mandelstam, 1997).

If major work is to be undertaken, the family needs to know whether they need plans drawn by an architect. They also need to know what planning permissions or building warrants are needed. It is advisable for the occupational therapist to work with the architect and family to ensure that dimensions drawn by the architect allow for any extra equipment or furniture that is to be used in the area (Clutton et al., 2006).

## FUNDING

The ownership of the house and the cost of the alterations determine who needs to be approached to help with funding. Some families may choose to fund the alterations by themselves (Bull, 1998). Each local authority area will have its own criteria and procedures for funding adaptations. The social work occupational therapist will be able to give advice about the funding processes in the local area.

The owner of the house can apply to the local council for a grant to make the house suitable for the person with Duchenne muscular dystrophy. A disabled person can also apply for the grant to alter their home to meet their needs, even if they are not the owner or the tenant, but the owner must agree to the grant application. Grants can be means tested (Office of the Deputy Prime Minister, 2002).

Many areas now have care-and-repair schemes (Scottish Homes, 1999a) that will help grant applicants through the process of getting costs for the adaptation prior to submitting the grant application. They can also be of great assistance in finding someone to supervise the project. It is vital that no work is started on the house before a grant application is made and approved by the council in writing. A grant will not be paid for any work already done.

Minor adaptations on owner–occupier properties can be funded by the local social services. In council-owned properties, it is the responsibility of the council to make the house suitable for the resident with Duchenne muscular dystrophy, assuming they have the budget resources. Housing associations also have to provide adaptations for their tenants. If it is a temporary adaptation, it may be the responsibility of the social services to fund the adaptation. The council and housing associations will normally only carry out the work needed following an assessment and recommendation from an occupational therapist (Scottish Homes, 1999b).

Some councils and housing associations may offer alternative housing to families rather than adapting their home, according to Oldman and Beresford (1998). This should only be considered if the family agree.

## FINDING A NEW HOUSE

Once the family have agreed that they wish to move house, there are three main options:

- to rent an alternative house;
- to buy another house;
- to build a house for the family.

The 'Housing Report' (Appendix VII) and the 'Housing Assessment' form (Appendix VIII) give details of what to look for when assessing the family's current housing situation. These reports can then be used to highlight the housing needs of the family to any housing providers. The report can also be used as a guide to the family for things they need to think about when viewing other properties that they are thinking of buying. It would be advisable to have the occupational therapist check any house that they are considering buying.

If the family need a purpose-built house, it can be useful to find out whether there are any new developments being planned in the area. Sometimes, the developers will consider building a house to the dimensions that the family need. This is usually a cheaper option and less time-consuming than having plans drawn, finding a plot and hiring a builder.

## EMOTIONAL ISSUES

Moving house or altering an existing house for a person with Duchenne muscular dystrophy is a very emotive situation.

Each alteration can highlight deterioration in the person's abilities. Sometimes, families delay in asking for alterations or equipment, as they are not ready to accept the decline in the person. When this happens, it is important to emphasise how the adaptation will benefit the person or their carer. If the family will not look ahead to future needs, this can lead to piecemeal adaptations that will deal with the immediate needs of the family but will not be suitable in the long term (Harpin, 2000). When this is done, each subsequent alteration can cause further anxieties for the family.

It is better to alter the housing situation to allow for all the future needs of the person with muscular dystrophy. Equipment should only be introduced when required.

Financing adaptations or moving house can be a major cause of anxiety for the family. They need to know how much they will have to contribute to the cost before making any decisions about their housing. Budget resources within local authorities can often mean the family have to find large sums of money before being able to proceed with major adaptations to their home (O'Brien, 2003). If the family cannot find this kind of money, it can cause stress within the family.

Any proposed alteration to the family home can upset the dynamics of the family, state Hawkins and Stewart (2002). Consideration has to be given to siblings' and parents' needs. Sometimes, the person with muscular dystrophy has to spend long periods of time in the bathroom; thus, another bathroom may be needed to provide facilities for others in the home. In many cases, compromises have to be worked out before any work is started, as the wishes of carers may oppose the wishes of the person with muscular dystrophy.

Parents of children with Duchenne muscular dystrophy have normally cared for their child since they were diagnosed. They can find it very hard when the child wants to leave home for university or to move into their own home. It takes a long time for each party to adjust to the proposed change. The young adult with muscular dystrophy should have control over who cares for them (Penson & Fisher, 1995). This can help to reduce embarrassment and improve their self-confidence.

Support is needed to find their way through the complexities of the adaptation processes and they need to feel in control of their own home. Offering practical assistance while the actual building work is being carried out can help to relieve stress within the household. Respite for all the family should be considered while major building work is disrupting the normal use of the house.

Good-quality adaptations can have a positive impact on the quality of life of the person and their family (Heywood, 2001). They can reduce stress within the family and can improve the health of the carer and the person with muscular dystrophy.

In the future, the need for major housing adaptations will disappear, as new building regulations should provide us with homes that are accessible to everyone (Audit Commission, 1998). It is unsuitable housing environments that make people disabled.

## KEY POINTS

- Consult all the family regarding their housing needs.
- Assess their existing house.
- Advise the family regarding adaptations that can be made in each room.
- Consider hazards and fire safety.
- Provide information on funding options for adaptations.
- If the house cannot be made accessible, explore housing alternatives acceptable to the family.
- Maximise family control in all housing decisions.

## CASE STUDY

The family lived in a recently built housing-association house. All the bed-rooms and the bathroom were upstairs in the house. There was a lounge, kitchen–diner and a downstairs toilet on the ground floor. All the doors were 900–925 mm wide, which was enough to allow wheelchair access between the rooms on each floor. There were three steps at the back and front doors to the house. The internal stairs blocked wheelchair access to the first floor. There was an enclosed garden to the back of the house and a small side and front garden with a driveway.

Following discussions with the family, it was established that they wished to stay in their present home but they were also aware that they could not continue to lift their child upstairs, as he was getting heavier. The child was being lifted up the stairs by his parents. This was placing the child and parents at risk.

There were three ways of overcoming the problem of lifting the child upstairs. The first was the provision of a lift. The second was the creation of a downstairs bedroom and toilet/shower room within the confines of the exist-ing building and the last was building an extension to the back of the house, providing a downstairs bedroom and bathroom for the child.

The child's mother fluctuated between accepting and rejecting the child's prognosis. This resulted in her opting for a series of staged adaptations rather than very radical alterations to the house. The family initially opted for the provision of a stair lift to carry the child upstairs but, once the child was too heavy to transfer on and off the stair lift, a downstairs bedroom and toilet/ shower room were provided.

A stair lift with postural support was provided at first, due to the vulnerabil-ity and young age of the child. He did not want to sleep alone downstairs. A bedroom on the ground floor would also have excluded him from being with the rest of the family at night. A through-the-floor lift was not an option, as too much bedroom and living space would be lost.

Subsequently, the child's mother developed back problems and consider-ation had to be given to providing a bathing and bedroom facility for the child on the ground floor. There was sufficient space on the ground floor to create a bedroom and install a tracking hoist. There was also an existing toilet down-stairs which, with some structural alterations, could be converted into a toilet/ shower room which would have adequate space for wheelchair access. This was the option that the family preferred.

Extending the building to provide a bedroom and bathroom facility was rejected by the family, as they would have lost most of the back garden, which was an important resource for the child and the family.

When the occupational therapist recommended the installation of a stair lift, she also recommended that a ramp be constructed at the back door of the house to allow wheelchair access from the street to the house. The family mainly entered the house via the back door. This door gave entrance to a large family kitchen where the child's mother spent most of her time during the day. The family wished the ramp to be placed at the back door, where it could not be seen from the street; they did not want the house to be seen as different. This was an acceptable option, as the child could be supervised and easily reached by family members in the kitchen while he was in the garden.

## STUDY QUESTIONS

- Name three ways in which a family can change their housing situation.
- If a stair lift cannot be installed in the house, what alternatives should be considered?
- What are piecemeal or staged adaptations?

# 13 Social Needs: An Overview

CLAIRE TESTER

## INTRODUCTION

All young children engage in play activities and play with peers. At nursery, the boy with Duchenne muscular dystrophy may be slower than other children in gross motor activities, and may fall more frequently, but he is to be actively encouraged and supported to play. The little boy may become aware of his difficulties and become frustrated with his own efforts. This should be handled sensitively and staff should not encourage the boy to try harder, as his frustration may develop. It is as the boy grows older and as the condition progresses that his proximal muscles affect his gross motor abilities and skills. In turn, this can affect the boy's ability to join in activities with his peers in the playground and games sessions at school. This can be isolating and depressing, depending upon how it is handled by the school staff, as there are ways in which the boy can be actively involved. Unfortunately, not all teaching staff are aware of how their own actions and words can affect the child. For example, class outings can exclude the boy: as one teacher remarked, 'We can't take you, you can't get on the bus for a start'. Considerations need to be made to be as inclusive as possible. In this way, the class take their cue from the staff, and may perceive that exclusion of the lad with Duchenne muscular dystrophy is acceptable. Bullying, too, in all its forms, needs to be addressed. Unfortunately, bullying can start with mocking behaviour, or not being included in playground activities. As boys often play football in break time, it renders the young man outside of the game. However, a whistle and a role as referee can make him active. This may require intervention by staff, and an active positive behaviour policy within the school is to be encouraged for all pupils. If there are signs of bullying which are not picked up by the staff, the boy needs to feel assured that he can discuss this with someone either at school or with his family. The Family Care Officer (FCO) employed by the Muscular Dystrophy Campaign, who visits and supports the family linking in with school, may be this person. Sometimes, the reaction to bullying can be aggressive behaviour on the part of the boy, or adolescent, using his chair to ram others, leading to getting himself into trouble and accused of bullying himself. Teaching staff benefit from support and practical guidance from a therapist. In this way, the occupational therapist may appear as an advocate for the young man. The Muscular Dystrophy Campaign (2004a) has produced a guide for teaching staff which is very helpful. The therapist may provide a copy for the school and for the parents, too, if the Family Care Officer from the Muscular Dystrophy Campaign has not already done so.

The question of who limits whom, and who reinforces a disability, needs to be asked at regular intervals as, unnecessarily, it may begin early in their life. For some young men, it is the people around them who make the decisions of what they can or cannot do. Chapter 3 covers some of the difficulties in social needs, but the stage after school needs to be considered, as this phase can be when young men get 'lost' and experience social deprivation (Bushby et al., 2001).

The young men who leave school at 16 years old and do not go onto higher education can quickly lose their daily social contact with their peers. The community physiotherapist and occupational therapist often provide a school-based service and this contact is lost. In addition, because school transport is provided on a daily basis, the young man becomes dependent upon his family to take him out. Depending upon his place in the family, for example, he may be the eldest child, whilst his siblings are at school and he is at home. As this young man is dependent for his needs, he needs help from another at home. For some parents, this is when a part-time job is given up in order to be at home with their son. This has financial implications and can curb activity further. This situation imposes restrictions which can result in a negative effect upon the mood and sense of purpose for the young man. Social networks and options to support social activities ideally need to be developed whilst at secondary school, which can be continued after school, both at weekends and on leaving school. The development of IT skills at school, with home internet access, is important but can be overlooked. An assessment of what is important and meaningful is necessary, which may involve the Model of Human Occupation (Kielhofner et al., 2002). The last year of school should be used to actively prepare and plan for school leaving. Continued contact should be made by the occupational therapist to support the family in practical ways, and to ensure a transition and referral to adult services (ACT, 2003).

There are different factors which affect the young man and how his social needs are met. These include the attitude of the boy about his own condition; his level of self-esteem and his own network of friends made at school and how these friendships are maintained; the attitude of his parents to support and encourage his friendships and social activity; the financial situation of the family in being able to fund social activities; the physical health and strength of the parents and family members in being able to assist in moving and handling manoeuvres and transfers required in transport; toileting in public toilets, etc. The local service provision for helpers/carers in dressing and bathing may be restricted to specific times for getting up in a morning and being 'put' to bed. All of these can compound the freedom that a young man might expect in his late teens. Understandably, some parents are protective of their sons and attempt to restrict activity, as this can tire the young man, who might need time to recover for the next day or two. This is a risk that many young men are willing to take. The element of risk is perhaps underestimated as being perceived as an essential part of youth. The additional difficulty of learning difficulties for some young men with Duchenne muscular dystrophy also compounds difficulties in developing a social life outside of the family.

Whilst some young men are supported to go out, to employ their own carers and have an active social life, others are sitting at home, seldom seeing anyone unless they visit the home. In turn, this can lead to depression and the associated loss of interest in life. This can create a sense of being a burden for the family. As these young men are in a transitional stage between children's and adults' services, regular monitoring for joint mobility, contractures, postural seating, including wheelchair, and activities of daily living are often not maintained. There can be a loss of contact with therapy services and an uncertainty by the family as to whom to contact. Families known to a children's hospice have contact with the therapists who will also refer them to community services. As social services act upon each referral and close the case without an ongoing review, the family needs to be aware of this. As discussed in Chapter 17, there is an identified need for support in social needs. Having recognised the social needs of the young man, how do restrictions and limitations in life occur? Are they inevitable? Problem-solving approaches need to be used, which can involve the family and school with the young man. This may take more time and effort but is worthwhile.

In thinking about the social needs and the associated independence required by these young men, it is helpful to consider what are the usual, normal experiences in adolescence. The following checklist identifies normal behaviour through early to late-stage adolescence as an overview.

## CHECKLIST

### EARLY ADOLESCENCE AT START OF PUBERTY INVOLVING 11, 12 AND 13 YEARS

- Friendships usually involving close friendships and company with one or two friends at a time.
- Development of secondary sexual characteristics, such as the growth of the body, pubic hair, change of voice, and voice breaking.
- Leads to comparison with peers and some anxiety, as some boys grow faster than others, or later onset of puberty; this can provoke feelings of not being normal, inadequacy.

- Embarrassment of the body and need for privacy.
- Lack of regard for the body in face of change, unwilling to wash regularly, hair combing, etc.
- Some regression in relationships with parents in face of change.
- Sexually functioning body becomes potent with adolescent's awareness of this; a reluctance to engage in parental intimacies, such as hand-holding, being hugged by mother, etc.
- Conflict with parent(s) in ideas, opinions, and can be disparaging of them.
- Shunning of being seen by peers with parent because of possible ridicule by them, 'Mummy's boy', etc.
- Degrees of separation from parent, wanting to be more independent, including shopping, social activities without parent intervention.
- Development of internal emotional life, no longer sharing thoughts and experiences with parent(s), development of emotional privacy.

## MID-TEENS FROM 14 TO 16 YEARS

- This may mark the onset of puberty, whilst, for peers, this may be well developed at this stage; there may be a prolonged immaturity because of this late onset, or worry that they are different and may not grow.
- Importance of friends/mates/peers usually as a member of a group.
- Aspect of mirroring peers becomes important; trying out different identities which can involve wearing same clothes, sharing same activities.
- Decision making and responsibility in choice of academic subjects, considering a future self and higher-education choices.
- Sense of failure/achievement relating to national examinations.
- Self-discipline and self-motivation in studying, working for school work and exams.
- Importance of role models in considering a possible future self.
- Saturday job or newspaper round leading to introduction to work and some independence with earning own money.
- Confidence in social skills, and self-esteem being worked upon.
- Physical and emotional attraction to another with internalised relationship.
- May be sexually active, but not always emotionally capable.
- Leaving childhood behind and outward signs relating to changing room posters, putting away/getting rid of toys; sense of awkwardness as can be in between these stages of moving towards adult life, and leaving aspects of known life behind; there can be uncertainty in how to address this stage by the adolescent.
- Time of experimentation with risk taking; this is carried through into late teens with alcohol, drugs, sexual experimentation.

## LATE ADOLESCENCE INVOLVING 17, 18 AND 19 YEARS, APPROACHING ADULTHOOD

- Preparation for leaving school or may have just left school.
- This can involve peers moving away and peer groups breaking up.
- Time of independence or preparing for independence.
- Full-time work and may be earning more money than peers.
- May be a time of unemployment and markedly less money than peers, possible lack of orientation.
- Higher education can incur student debt and financial as well as academic pressure.
- Sexual relationships.
- By late adolescence, a stability of self-identity, reaching a sense of security in own identity as a young adult.

The purpose of the checklist is to refer to it as a guide for normal adolescence and to be aware of any restrictions which may be imposed unintentionally by others upon a young man with Duchenne muscular dystrophy. This should be handled sensitively with both parents and the young man.

## COMMENT

Whilst there are individual differences, these are broadly the same experiences in travelling through adolescence. These involve identity formation, sexual identity, physical development and physical growth. Adolescence is marked by an enormous period of change and increasing independence which needs to be recognised and supported by the parent(s). The family attitude toward the growing adolescent impacts on the development; for example, if he is the youngest sibling, the family may regard the adolescent as the 'baby' of the family, which can be a difficult perception, even as an adult. The role models available in the family, including the extended family, have an affect, too. For example, if parents are unemployed or in full-time work, this can shape the thinking of what it means to be an adult in this family. Some parents have difficulty in perceiving their children as capable, independent individuals, which can lead to real conflict or an enforced passivity.

In considering this checklist for adolescence, it should be balanced with any learning or behavioural difficulties, and an awareness of potential conflict in the family if a young man has a sense of being thwarted in his development as a person. Problem solving may be required in considering aspects of normal adolescent activity. For example, grandparents or parents of close friends who may want to include the young man for evening meals or even sleep-overs would find it helpful to have the advice of an occupational therapist in assessing and identifying needs which can be simple. In one such situation, the young man and his friends at a 'sleepover' all slept downstairs, watching a late-night film. A portable ramp was used for the front door, and a urinal sheath used, as well as a small portable hoist for toileting purposes with practical teaching. Portable ramps and a rearrangement of furniture are small but significant changes. One 18-year-old with Duchenne muscular dystrophy commented that he was going to be spending Christmas Day at home alone, with phone calls and visits from his older brother, as his family were planning to be at his grandparents for the day. He could not go, as there was no ramp or small portable hoist.

Adolescence, which is considered stretching through the teenage years until reaching 20, is a crucial and formative period in one's life, entering as a child and, hopefully, leaving as an independent, responsible and capable adult. In considering an adolescent with Duchenne muscular dystrophy, these stages are just as important but the condition affects body image and confidence, and results in increasing physical dependence. Being washed, toileted, dressed and undressed by others who may be parents or carers employed by local services can be embarrassing for the adolescent. As one young man commented, 'These are usually ladies in their fifties who chat over me and are in a hurry to be off to someone else. I have to go to bed at the time they can come in the evening.' Also, physical dependence upon others for activities of daily living is increasing. This increasing dependence as the young man reaches his mid-teens is in opposition to the independence of his peers at the same age. The emotional and developmental needs of the young man with Duchenne muscular dystrophy should be recognised. These must also be considered in the light of any learning difficulties. A further conflict can arise when parents can find it difficult to let their son lead an increasingly independent life when their worries and concerns increase as he gets older (see Chapter 3).

## KEY POINTS

- Besides physical development, there is emotional development, too.
- Adolescence is an important time for friendships and developing independence.
- Adolescence can be described as formative, as it prepares for adulthood.
- Learning difficulties may present with an emotional immaturity.
- The social needs of someone with Duchenne muscular dystrophy are important to consider in line with what is 'normal' and appropriate.

## CASE STUDY

Brian's parents can no longer undertake all of the tasks of activities of daily living for Brian, and carers are to attend Brian every morning. Brian is 12. He is reluctant to have anyone wash, toilet and dress him. His parents cannot see another option. He has become argumentative with his parents and refuses to cooperate in anything with them.

What might Brian be angry about? How might the situation be improved?

## STUDY QUESTIONS

- Consider someone approaching puberty, who also has Duchenne muscular dystrophy. What are the difficulties that he is facing?
- Consider someone aged 15 years old with Duchenne muscular dystrophy. What might he be experiencing?
- Consider someone aged 19 years of age who has Duchenne muscular dystrophy. What might this young man be considering?

These three questions may be applied to someone with learning difficulties and to someone without any learning difficulties.

# 14 Employment

KATE STONE

## INTRODUCTION

As people with Duchenne muscular dystrophy are living longer, employment has become more of an issue for these young men. This chapter will look at ways to prepare people for employment and what services are available to help them. It will also consider their employment rights and ways to fund any adjustments that are needed for them to start or continue to work.

Planning for employment for boys with muscular dystrophy, as with other young people, should start when they are at school. Parental attitudes can have a great influence on their children's educational and employment aspirations. Young people with good social skills, attractive personalities and good qualifications have better employment opportunities than those who do not have these attributes.

Children need to select subjects that they find motivating and stimulating that could lead to careers that they can pursue. Some young men will choose to attend further education to enhance their qualifications, but they also need to be realistic in the courses that they select if they plan to use them as a basis for employment. These courses can be at specialist colleges or mainstream colleges or universities. The university they select can also influence their employment potential, as qualifications from some establishments are more valued by potential employers.

The introduction of disability discrimination legislation and advances in medical science, technology and flexible working practices now make employment a reality for people with Duchenne muscular dystrophy.

## OCCUPATIONAL THERAPISTS AND WORK

Developing a vocational identity is an important part of adolescent development, regardless of their health status. Occupational therapists can have a role in fostering vocational readiness in boys with Duchenne muscular dystrophy by encouraging them to talk about what they want to do when they are older. They can also raise the subject of the boy's expectations regarding employment, as well as establishing what their parents' and their teachers' views are of the boy's work prospects. This will ensure that everyone has a realistic view of his future employment possibilities and will hopefully raise their expectations. It is not uncommon for people to have low expectations of these boys' working in any capacity. The occupational therapist should also be able to provide advice on agencies that can help with career advice and further-education choices. The therapist should also encourage the boy to seek work experiences while he is still at school in order to develop links with possible employers (Shaw et al., 2006).

Rehabilitation for work is a duty that occupational therapists often share with the employment services. Employment services are constantly changing, as is legislation; therefore, occupational therapists need to keep up to date with the current situation when dealing with work-related issues (Silcox, 2003).

Occupational therapists can also offer practical help in suggesting adaptations to the workplace and work methods to enable the individual to carry out their job. The Pathways to Work – an NHS and Jobcentre partnership scheme – also employs occupational therapists along with other health professionals to help people claiming benefits to get into work (Department of Work and Pensions, 2002).

Therapists also need to be aware of the different funding sources and support agencies that can assist a young man with Duchenne muscular dystrophy to gain and sustain employment.

## CAREERS ADVICE

Before a young man with Duchenne muscular dystrophy can apply for any job, he needs to get some careers advice. Most boys will have access to a careers adviser at school and, if they go on to university, they can access career advice services there. They can also access the university careers advice centres for up to three years after they have left university. Career advisers or the Connexions service, which provides advice to the 13–19 age group, can assist the individual to work out what educational courses they wish to take with a view to the sort of employment that they are seeking. The service can also provide information on ways into the career of their choice and can give information on the content of courses and how courses can be funded. They can also help with transition plans for youths with Duchenne muscular dystrophy while they are still at school (Connexions, 2006).

Finding the right career is a matter of matching personality, skills and interests to a job that will best suit the needs and aspirations of the individual. Therefore, a boy with Duchenne muscular dystrophy needs to identify what he is good at academically, what subjects he enjoys and why he enjoys them. He should also consider what hobbies he likes and why he gets satisfaction from them. Consideration should also be given to the type of environment he likes to be in. Does he prefer noise or quiet, working with others or working alone? This is the basis for identifying a career that he may be interested in pursuing. Prior to deciding on a particular course, it is advisable to talk to a lot of people about the work they do. Where possible, a visit to different working environments can be initiated long before the boy leaves school (Skill: National Bureau for Students with Disabilities, 2006).

There are a number of ways to get support to gain employment. Most of them can be accessed via disability employment advisers, who can be contacted at job centres. There are a number of strategies for accessing employment but none is universally applicable to all disabled workers. People with Duchenne muscular dystrophy will have to have some idea of their goals and expectations when seeking employment and they should also consider what type of basic assistance they will need at work.

## DISABILITY EMPLOYMENT ADVISERS

Disability employment advisers offer support to people with a disability who have problems getting employment or those who think they may lose their job due to their disability. They can give support to help find work or to access training that could lead to work. In order to work out the best way in which they can give support, they will normally carry out an employment assessment.

## EMPLOYMENT ASSESSMENTS

An employment assessment helps to find out what skills a person with Duchenne muscular dystrophy can bring to an employer. It may also identify skills that have to be developed to improve the person's employment opportunities. The assessment will also discuss the types of work that the person is interested in obtaining and how their medical condition may influence their choice of work. At the end of the assessment, an action plan should be drawn up, setting goals towards achieving employment.

## WORKSTEP

WORKSTEP is another government scheme that supports disabled people who have more complex problems to overcome to get a job. It provides support to the individual and the employer tailored to the person's needs. An individual plan is created that allows the person to develop their skills. This may be via job tasters, work experience or training with a view to obtaining work.

## NEW DEAL FOR DISABLED PEOPLE

This is another scheme that helps to match people with employers through training and skill development. It also helps the individual through the process of applying for jobs and will provide support through the first six months in work (Jobcentreplus, 2007b).

## JOB INTRODUCTION SCHEME

The Job Introduction Scheme can help an employer and the person with muscular dystrophy to discover whether a job suits the individual. This scheme will help to decide whether the person with muscular dystrophy can cope in the working environment and will also give the employer a chance to ascertain whether the individual can cope with work.

The Job Introduction Scheme can help by paying a grant to the employer for the first few weeks that will help with costs. This Scheme can be accessed via the disability employment advisers but it must be applied for before starting work. There are certain criteria that need to be met to qualify for the Job Introduction Scheme (Enable Together, 2007).

## ACCESS TO WORK

Access to Work is a government scheme that gives assistance to disabled people at work. It can provide funding for additional support needs related to their employment that can help a person with muscular dystrophy to work. It will fund the following:

• support for personal care and some work tasks;
• equipment to help with personal care at work and employment activities;
• adaptations to the building or workstations;
• additional transport costs to work or within working hours;
• communication support at interviews.

A 100% funding is available for people starting work and the funding approved will last for three years, after which it will be reviewed. To obtain a full grant for costs, the application must be made within six weeks of starting work.

These are the basic government schemes that can be accessed to help with employment issues. The disability employment adviser usually determines which scheme would best meet the individual's needs (Brading & Curtis, 1996).

## THE NEUROMUSCULAR CENTRE

Other training schemes are available through a variety of voluntary organisations. One of the most relevant agencies for people with Duchenne muscular dystrophy is the Neuromuscular Centre, which is part of the Muscular Dystrophy Campaign. This centre provides training, work opportunities and treatment for people with muscular dystrophy. They also provide transport and support services for individuals attending the centre. Within the centre, there is a graphic design and print company, which is run by and employs people with muscular dystrophy (Neuromuscular Centre, 2007).

## DISABILITY DISCRIMINATION ACT 1995

People with Duchenne muscular dystrophy have the same employment rights as others and their rights were strengthened with the introduction of the Disability Discrimination Act 1995. This Act makes it unlawful to discriminate against disabled people for a reason that is connected to their disability. This covers all the following aspects of recruitment and employment:

- job advertisements;
- application forms;
- interviews;
- terms of employment;
- training opportunities;
- promotion opportunities;
- dismissal.

This Act also puts a duty on employers to make reasonable changes to the workplace or the way in which the work is completed to assist the disabled person to work. Examples of these are:

- adaptations to the building to provide access or toilet facilities;
- flexible working hours to allow for health appointments;
- modifying working equipment;
- changing work locations to allow access;
- providing training;
- allocating some of the disabled person's duties to others;
- modifying instructions or software.

The law requires all companies to make reasonable adjustments for people with disabilities, unless doing so would impose an undue hardship on the company. All adjustments need to be suited to the individual's needs and the essential functions of the particular job (Cooper & Vernon, 1996).

## EMPLOYERS

Some employers are more committed to employing people with a disability than others. This is worth remembering when looking for employment. The 'two ticks' disability symbol is awarded to companies or organisations that have taken positive steps towards employing disabled people. They display this symbol on their job adverts. However, applications should still be made to any company or organisation if the job advertised appears to suit the individual. One cannot predict how any company will react to an application from a person with Duchenne muscular dystrophy who has the qualifications and potential to fill the post advertised.

Organisations are more likely to offer employment to people with muscular dystrophy, especially if they have regular contact with this group.

Employers often have other good reasons for employing people with a disability. They generally stay in a job longer and are more committed to their work. They can also be a stimulus to encourage more disabled people to be customers of the company (Employment–Solicitors, 2007).

There are ways of working other than the traditional idea of applying for a job with a company and working at the company's base. The New Deal scheme also allows people the opportunity to set up their own business. Some people choose to work freelance from home, doing work such as web design, accountancy and writing. When considering this option, some thought has to be given as to whether they will operate as a self-employed sole trader, a limited company or through an umbrella company, as this may have a substantial effect on benefit entitlements.

There are many ways in which to search for a job, including some specialised websites for disabled people, but the important issue is to keep looking for job opportunities by any method – volunteering, career fairs or information from friends can be just as effective a way of finding the right job as any other.

## INTERVIEWS

It is up to the individual with Duchenne muscular dystrophy as to when they decide to tell a potential employer about their medical condition. Normally, it is advisable to inform them prior to interview to allow them to make suitable arrangements. The Access to Work scheme can also provide help to get a person with muscular dystrophy to an interview.

During an interview, the focus should be on the skills and abilities that the person with Duchenne muscular dystrophy can bring to the job. The individual should not be reluctant to ask what opportunities the job will bring them. It is also good to research the philosophy of the company, as many companies are more proactive in supporting people with disabilities than others. However, it is advisable for the person with muscular dystrophy to be prepared with solutions on how to make adjustments to the workplace to allow them to be competent in the job. It also helps to offer suggestions on how to fund these adjustments, as employers are not always aware of schemes like Access to Work (Skill: National Bureau for Students with Disabilities, 2006).

## WORK ADJUSTMENTS

The following are a number of different work adjustments that are recommended for people with muscular dystrophy by Batiiste (2005):

- a personal-care assistant at work;
- provide access to the workplace and to the toilet areas near the person's workstation;
- allow breaks away from the workstation;
- flexible working to allow for health appointments;
- allow working from home;
- modify workstation to meet the individual's needs, such as computer access, telephone adaptations, mobile arm supports and book supports;
- parking near the workplace;
- train other staff regarding the individual's needs.

Each job and individual will have different adjustments that will have to be considered. A balance has to be reached as to what is reasonable for the company and what is not. Some adjustments may make it impossible for other employees to carry out their work.

## DISCRIMINATION

Legislation has made it illegal to discriminate against a disabled person with regard to employment but this does not mean that it does not happen. Care needs to be taken to ensure the discrimination is because of the disability and not for some other reason – some people can believe they did not get a job or were passed over for promotion because of their disability but, in reality, it may be because they do not have the best qualifications or their work performance was poor.

However, when a person feels they are being discriminated against because of their disability, they should raise the issue with the employer to see whether it can be resolved. If this fails, the Disability Rights Commission can give detailed guidance to both the employer and the employee regarding resolving the situation or lodging a complaint (Disability Rights Commission, 2007).

## FLEXIBLE WORKING FOR CARERS

The Employment Act 2002 gives carers of a disabled child of less than 18 years of age the right to ask for flexible working hours. Employers need to consider such a request but they are able to refuse under certain conditions. The government also has plans to make flexible working available to all carers (Dimond, 2004).

## KEY POINTS

- It is possible for a person with Duchenne muscular dystrophy to gain employment.
- Plan and consider career options while the boy is still in school.
- Expose the person to working environments and the work ethic.
- There are many ways to get help to access employment.
- Workplaces and work methods can be altered.
- Understand employment rights, especially the Disability Discrimination Act 1995.

## CASE STUDY

Graduating from university with a degree in accounting, a young man with Duchenne muscular dystrophy obtained a position in a bank. The young man required funding and assistance to take up his post. He approached his local authority occupational therapist to find out what services and funding were available to assist him to get to his work and to deal with personal-care issues at work. The occupational therapist completed a community-care assessment which identified the young man's needs and developed a care plan for the individual, but, in an effort to speed up the funding and resources process, a case conference was arranged. The young man, his parents, a representative from the bank and all the agencies that could provide support or resources to allow the young man to commence his employment were invited.

The representative from the bank agreed to find a suitable work location on the ground floor of the bank near the occupational health employment suite. That had accommodation where his personal-care needs could be met. The young man needed enough care to qualify for funding from the

Independent Living Fund. The representative from this service agreed to help the young man employ his own personal assistants who would assist him at work and home and would transport him to and from work.

The costs for the personal assistant were to be split between funding from the Independent Living Scheme and the Access to Work Scheme. The Access to Work Scheme also agreed to fund a special keyboard and a hands-free telephone for the young man to use at work and to modify the entrance door that the young man would use to access the bank.

## STUDY QUESTIONS

- What costs could the Access to Work scheme cover?
- How can a disability employment adviser help to find work?
- What right do people with Duchenne muscular dystrophy have under the Disability Discrimination Act 1995?
- Name three adjustments that would assist a person with Duchenne muscular dystrophy to work.
- What rights do carers have under the Employment Act 2002?

# 15 Transport

KATE STONE

## INTRODUCTION

Transport is vital to children and adults with Duchenne muscular dystrophy. They need transport to access education, hospitals, employment and leisure pursuits. The type of transport needed will change over the course of their illness and the methods of transport used will vary to meet their travel needs. Occupational therapists will often be involved in assessments relating to the transport requirements of people with Duchenne muscular dystrophy. They also need to know how to assist individuals onto different forms of transport, as they often accompany individuals on outings. Occupational therapists are often responsible for organising transport for people with muscular dystrophy to attend treatment or leisure activities, so they should be aware of their transport requirements.

Initially, when a child starts to have mobility problems, he will have to rely on different methods of transport to get him about his home and to other locations. He may need a wheelchair or buggy to allow him to accompany his family when they are out walking or he may require a taxi or a bus to get him to school.

While a child is using a manual wheelchair for mobility, he may be able to transfer in and out of an ordinary car but, once he is using a powered wheelchair to move about his environment, he will normally need to travel in a car or van that has a ramp or a lift (Campbell et al., 2000). The vehicle used has to suit the person with Duchenne muscular dystrophy, their family or carer and their wheelchair.

## DISABILITY LIVING ALLOWANCE

This is an important benefit that can assist people with care and transport costs in the UK. Children or adults with Duchenne muscular dystrophy who are permanent residents in the UK will normally qualify for this benefit once they reach the age of three.

Occupational therapists can be of assistance in obtaining and filling in application forms for the Disability Living Allowance and they are often asked to supply reports to support applications for people applying for this benefit.

Qualifying for the high-rate mobility component of this benefit opens the door to other benefits and services. People on the high-rate mobility component of the Disability Living Allowance can access the Motability Scheme.

## MOTABILITY SCHEME

Motability is a charity set up to assist disabled people with their transport needs. The Motability scheme can assist people with Duchenne muscular dystrophy to obtain powered wheelchairs and cars using their mobility allowances. It also administers government grants for people who need complex car adaptations and wheelchair-accessible vehicles.

When considering complex car adaptations or buying expensive powered wheelchairs or cars, it is advisable to seek good information. This can be obtained from reputable dealers recommended by the Motability scheme and from mobility centres that are located throughout the UK. These centres offer advice on all aspects of transport and can provide detailed assessments that help with the selection of appropriate vehicles and vehicle adaptations.

The Motability scheme can also help with the cost of driving lessons for young people or a nominated person to drive them if they are not able to drive or do not wish to drive (Motability, 2007).

## ROAD TAX

People with muscular dystrophy on the higher-rate mobility component of the Disability Living Allowance are exempt from paying road tax, even if they are not the driver of the car – providing the car is mainly used for their transport needs (Directgov, 2007a).

## PARKING BADGES AND PARKING BAYS

Local authorities administer the Blue Parking Badge Scheme, but the badge is valid throughout the UK and the European Union. Anyone on the high-rate mobility component of the Disability Living Allowance can obtain a parking badge, but there may be a small charge. Parking badges are issued automatically if you are on the high-rate mobility component. However, they can be issued following an assessment for people who do not qualify under the automatic criteria.

It is advisable to obtain a parking badge as soon as possible, as it can be of great benefit in helping to get parked nearer locations, especially hospitals. More and more hospitals require the display of a parking badge to be able to park in the hospital car parks.

The parking badge allows free use of on-street parking bays that are normally subject to parking charges. It may also allow extended parking times in the parking bays. There are two types of disabled parking bays: those enforceable by law and parking bays that are not legally enforceable.

Many parking bays provided for specific people outside their home are not enforceable due to the time it takes to make parking bays legally enforceable. Check with the local authority which type of parking bay they provide for individuals. Each local authority has criteria for providing parking bays.

Local authority occupational therapists are able to supply information on the procedures for obtaining parking badges and parking bays and may be involved in assessments relating to the provision of both.

Parking bays within hospitals, stores, railway stations and airports are operated by the owners of the car parks. They decide the costs and criteria for parking in their car parks (Directgov, 2007b).

## TRANSPORT TO HOSPITAL

There are different ways that assistance can be given to help attend hospital appointments. The local hospital trust can organise an ambulance, a hospital car or a taxi to attend appointments should your level of mobility warrant the need for transport. Help with the cost of travel to hospital and for overnight accommodation can also be provided through the Hospital Travel Cost Scheme. Accommodation costs will only be met if it is required to be able to attend appointments.

This scheme is available to people on low incomes, especially those in receipt of Income Support and Child and Working Tax Credits. If escorts are needed to accompany the person attending hospital, their costs will also be met by this scheme. If car-parking charges have to be paid at the hospital, these can also be claimed back under the Hospital Travel Cost Scheme (Department of Health, 2005).

A Community Care Grant can be given from the Social Fund to help with the costs of visiting someone in hospital but this is a discretionary grant and strict criteria have to be met before it will be awarded.

## TRANSPORT TO SCHOOLS AND NURSERIES

The education service of the local authority is responsible for providing transport to school and nursery for children with additional support needs, which include children with Duchenne muscular dystrophy. Each local authority will have its own policy regarding the provision of free transport to a school or nursery. If they agree to provide free transport, the vehicle used must meet the needs of the person whom they are transporting and must be fitted with any equipment that they need, such as a ramp or a lift. They are also responsible for providing an escort who is aware of the child's needs. Transport for school or nursery trips and after-school clubs at school should also be provided (Audit Commission, 2007).

## TRANSPORT TO FURTHER EDUCATION

Several organisations can be involved in providing funding for transport to universities and colleges of further education. Under the Education Act 1996, local authorities need to ensure that disabled students are not disadvantaged from attending further education due to transport difficulties and, under the Disability Discrimination Act 1995, institutions are also required to make reasonable adjustments to ensure that disabled students can study at the same level as non-disabled students. One of these adjustments could include the provision of additional transport costs.

Social services as well as education services can also assist with funding transport to further education courses under the Chronically Sick and Disabled Persons Act 1970, but assistance may not be available if resources are limited.

Each local authority, university and college can provide information on the different sources of funding for transport costs. Funding sources for transport costs vary across Britain and the funding sources can be different for different courses. However, if a student is in receipt of the higher-rate mobility component of the Disability Living Allowance, colleges and universities will take this into consideration when considering transport costs (Waters, 2006).

## TRANSPORT TO EMPLOYMENT

Through the Access to Work programme, there is funding for any additional travel costs for a disabled person and this may also include funding for a companion. Most people will be expected to use the mobility component of their Disability Living Allowance to cover the costs of getting to work (Jobcentreplus, 2007a).

## TRAVEL BY PRIVATE CAR

Gaining access to a vehicle is a necessity for people with Duchenne muscular dystrophy at all stages of their illness. There are a variety of methods available that can help to get the person and their wheelchair into vehicles.

In the early stages of their illness, a child will be able to transfer in and out of the car independently but they may need a car seat to provide good postural support while they are travelling. Before purchasing any car seat, it is important to try the seat to make sure it provides the postural support that the child needs. It is also important to make sure that the seat can be fitted safely into the cars used to transport the child. There are some harnesses on the market that can be fitted in a car to give more postural support. When using this type of harness, the seatbelt must be fastened. There are different harnesses for different models of car, so always make sure the harness is the right model for the car that the person is using, as it is dangerous to use the wrong harness.

Car seats for older children and special-needs car seats tend to be heavier, so make sure that the parents or carers can lift the car seat in and out of the car easily if it has to be removed from the car on a regular basis. Some special-needs seats have permanent fixings to secure them to the car that make it difficult to move them between vehicles. Other special-needs car seats can swivel 90° to make it easier to transfer in and out of the car and some can assist with sit-to-stand transfers for children with Duchenne muscular dystrophy who can still stand.

While the child is able to sit in a car seat, they will still have to store and transport their wheelchair. Their carer may be able to lift the wheelchair in and out of the vehicle but, if they are not able to do so, there are a variety of wheelchair hoists that can be fitted on the rear, side or roof of the car. Some hoists can only be used to lift folded manual wheelchairs, so check that any hoist proposed would lift the child's wheelchair and that it can be fitted into the car. When considering a hoist installation, also check that there will still be enough space in the car for the family.

Once the person with Duchenne muscular dystrophy cannot transfer into a car seat, they will have to access the vehicle sitting in their wheelchair. There are car hoists which can hoist people in and out of cars but, normally, the person has to be able to bend their head and lift their legs to get into the car. They are not a good method of accessing a car for a person with Duchenne muscular dystrophy, especially those who have had their spine fixed.

It is advisable to use a wheelchair-accessible vehicle, which is one in which the driver or a passenger can access the vehicle sitting in their wheelchair. If considering this type of vehicle, there needs to be sufficient headroom for the person sitting in the wheelchair. A head rest should be fitted to the wheelchair to reduce the risk of whiplash injuries and the chair should be properly fixed to the vehicle with a safety belt fixed to the car to keep the person safely in their wheelchair while travelling. On long journeys, it is hard to maintain an upright posture in a wheelchair. If the person's wheelchair has a tilt-in-space facility, this can make the journey more comfortable. It is recommended that the wheelchair used in the car has been crash-tested for use in a vehicle (Muscular Dystrophy Campaign, 2006).

Access to this type of vehicle is via a lift or a ramp. Some ramps need to be clipped onto the vehicle, which means that they have to be lifted into place. This type of ramp is not ideal if there are many transfers every day, as carers have enough physical tasks to perform. The effort involved in taking a person out should always be minimised to ensure that getting out does not become an arduous task.

When using a lift to access cars, make sure that it is the right size for the wheelchair being used and that it is designed to take the weight of the wheelchair with the person sitting in the chair.

Everyone who will be assisting the person with muscular dystrophy to access their vehicle must be properly trained in how to operate the ramp or lift that gives access to the vehicle. They also need to know how to position the person and their wheelchair in the vehicle to make certain that both are properly secured before any journey is started (Ricability, 2005).

## TRAVEL BY TAXI

Everyone has times when they cannot use their own transport, so it is important to be able to access alternative methods of transport. One of the most convenient are taxis, which can offer transport from door to door.

More and more taxi firms can provide wheelchair-accessible taxis. However, it is wise to check the size of wheelchair that they can accommodate before booking the taxi, as some wheelchair-accessible taxis cannot accommodate powered wheelchairs. The taxi-licensing office at the local council can advise on companies who have wheelchair-accessible taxis. Most 'black cabs' in London and larger cities are wheelchair-accessible but, again, they may not be accessible for people using larger powered wheelchairs. Never travel sideways in a taxi or any other vehicle, as it is not safe, and always make sure that the wheelchair brakes are on and that the power is switched of in powered wheelchairs while in the taxi, for safety.

## TRAVEL BY BUS

Access to buses is becoming easier for people in Britain who use wheelchairs, as all new buses have to be wheelchair-accessible but it will still be some time before all buses can accommodate wheelchairs. The new low-floor buses are also beneficial for children with Duchenne muscular dystrophy, as they eliminate the need to negotiate steps to get in and out of the bus.

Public service wheelchair-accessible buses have set spaces, which have been designed for transporting people in wheelchairs. Wheelchair users must use these spaces for their safety and the safety of other passengers.

Coaches used for long-distance travel generally are not wheelchair-accessible but, like other bus services, they are slowly changing to provide wheelchair-accessible buses on some routes. Even if there is access for a wheelchair user at present, coaches generally do not have toilets that are wheelchair-accessible.

Make certain when travelling by coach or on any long-distance journeys that everything that the person travelling in their wheelchair requires during the journey is accessible, such as food and medication. Always check with the coach operators what facilities and assistance are available at the coach stations and on the coaches before booking. It is also sensible to check how to access and exit the coach stations, as all entrances may not be wheelchair-accessible.

Some companies still need to know in advance that a wheelchair user is travelling on the coach and they also need to know ahead if folded wheelchairs have to be stored on the coaches. Hopefully, as access to all methods of transport improves, it will not be necessary to book any public transport in advance.

There are a growing number of companies that hire out wheelchair-accessible coaches for group outings or holidays and there are Dial a Bus services throughout the UK that offer door-to-door services for people with disability problems.

There are many types of bus services and bus operators in Britain but, in general, when a person with Duchenne muscular dystrophy is travelling on a bus sitting in a wheelchair, the wheelchair should always be positioned on the bus facing forward or rearward. It is dangerous to be positioned sideways. When travelling, it is safer to have a head support fitted to the wheelchair, as it reduces the risk of whiplash injuries if there is a crash. The wheelchair needs to be secured before travelling and the person in the wheelchair should also have diagonal and full harness restraint to keep them in position. These restraints should be anchored to the bus. Young men who have had their spine fixed should ideally have a full harness fitted to ensure that they can maintain a midline position when travelling and the harness will prevent them from falling forward. They should never travel with just a lap strap securing them in place.

Wheelchair access to the bus should always be via the rear or nearside of the bus. This is usually by a ramp or a lift. Bus access ramps should be a minimum of 800 mm wide and have a non-slip surface (Disabled Persons Transport Advisory Committee, 2001).

## TRAVEL BY FERRIES AND SHIPS

Just as it is important to check facilities and access to coach stations, the same checks have to be carried out for ports and dock areas where ferries or ships are boarded. Make sure that there are adequate toilet and catering facilities in the terminal buildings, as there can often be delays in accessing ferries and ships due to weather conditions.

Ports can be vast, so check the distance that has to be covered on foot or in a wheelchair from the nearest drop-off point to the ship. If this is a long distance, ascertain whether alternative methods of transport are offered for travelling within the port boundaries. Facilities at ports differ within the UK and abroad, so check what is offered at every port on the journey.

Ferries and cruise ships are operated by a number of companies, so check with the individual company before booking what services and facilities they can offer. Some companies have policies that require disabled people to be escorted.

Vessels vary. Modern ferries and ships will be wheelchair-accessible, with accessible cabins, toilet facilities and lifts between decks, but, as with other forms of transport, there are still older ferries and ships that are not wheelchair-accessible. Therefore, make sure that the company knows what type of access is needed so they can advise whether the vessel can meet the needs of the person travelling.

Consideration has to be given as to how to get on board a ferry. If access is via a vehicle and you need to get off the car deck, try to arrange for the vehicle to be parked near a lift that gives access to the other decks. Getting on board walking or using a wheelchair may not be a problem but some access ramps can be very steep. If this is the case, it may be possible to access the vessel via the car deck.

When planning a cruise, make certain all the public areas as well as the cabin facilities will accommodate the person travelling as well as their companions. Remember to check the bathing facilities and that the beds will also meet their needs. People who use powered wheelchairs need to check there is access to a power point to charge their wheelchairs. Oxygen users will have to check whether a supply is available on board the ship.

## TRAVEL BY TRAIN

When travelling by train, make sure that there is access to the train for a person in a wheelchair at the stations and that they and their wheelchair can be accommodated on the train, as some larger wheelchairs do not fit inside standard trains. Some older stations are not accessible and it may be necessary to choose different departure and arrival stations, which have better access. Station staff may have to escort you onto the trains via routes other than those used by mobile passengers. They may also have to put ramps in place for you to enter and exit the trains. Until all stations and trains are accessible, it is still necessary to book assistance to get on the train in advance. However, if you travel on the train on a regular basis, this may not be necessary.

Information is available from National Rail enquires regarding access to specific stations. On longer journeys, check that there are accessible toilets and catering facilities. The Eurostar service is accessible for wheelchair users but check that other European rail services are accessible before travelling (National Rail, 2006).

# TRAVEL BY UNDERGROUND

People using a wheelchair cannot use the majority of the underground railway systems, although some of the more modern lines do have wheelchair access. There is an access guide for the London underground that gives details of stations that can be accessed avoiding stairs or escalators.

# TRAVEL BY TRAM

The modern tram systems throughout the country are wheelchair-accessible but it is advisable to check whether they can accommodate larger powered wheelchairs.

# TRAVEL BY AEROPLANE

Airlines have different polices, services and charges for people who are wheel-chair users. It is vital to check out what each airline offers before booking a seat. Check that the airports, aeroplanes and toilet areas used at each stage of the journey are accessible. Remember that aircrew are not allowed to assist with toileting (Disabled Living Foundation, 1994). Plans for transferring onto the plane and transfers from the airport to the holiday accommodation need to be detailed to make sure that they meet the needs of all the people travelling in the party.

Most people with Duchenne muscular dystrophy will have to check the seating that is available on the plane, as they will often need postural support. Airlines can deal with seating requests as long as they have advance warning. Most airlines will carry mobility equipment free and can offer an oxygen supply during long trips, if requested.

# CONCESSIONARY FARES

## BUSES

People on the higher or middle rate of the Disability Living Allowance resident in Scotland are entitled to free bus travel on local and long-distance buses throughout Scotland. A National Entitlement Card is needed to access this service; these are available from the local authority. A Companion Concessionary Card is available through this scheme to allow a companion to travel free to assist on the journey (Transport Scotland, 2007).

In England, the entitlement is for free off-peak local travel, but if you live in Wales, free bus travel is available at any time of day. Bus passes are available from the local authority. In Northern Ireland, there is half-price travel for people in receipt of the mobility component of the Disability Living Allowance through the Smart Pass scheme.

On long-distance coach journeys between Scotland, England and Wales, you can get half-price tickets with some companies.

## TRAINS

The disabled person's rail card entitles a person with muscular dystrophy and a companion to one-third off the price of the rail ticket in England, Scotland and Wales. There is a charge for this card. However, a wheelchair user who has to travel on the train sitting in their wheelchair is also entitled to ticket concessions for themselves and a companion without the disabled person's rail card. In Northern Ireland, the person with muscular dystrophy can travel for half the price of the rail ticket using the Smart Card scheme.

## FERRIES

Each ferry company has its own policy regarding concessionary fares for disabled passengers. Contact the company to find out what concessions they offer; some do not offer any concessions.

## TAXIS

Many areas of the UK operate taxi voucher schemes for disabled people who cannot use public transport.

## AIRLINES

Airlines in general do not offer concessionary fares to disabled travellers.

## ASSISTANCE DOGS

Most forms of public transport in the UK allow assistance dogs such as dogs for the disabled to travel free, but they may have specific requirements that have to be adhered to before the dog can travel.

## ESCORTS

As discussed before, there are some concessionary fares available for companions and escorts who accompany an individual with Duchenne muscular dystrophy. The Red Cross can also provide escorts and suitable transport for individuals and families. There is usually a charge for this service (British Red Cross, 2007).

# WHEELCHAIRS

Wheelchairs are essential forms of transport for people with Duchenne muscular dystrophy; they need them to participate in everyday life when they have difficulty walking. They will need different types of wheelchairs at different stages in their illness. When selecting a wheelchair, get good advice about what is available and about how it can be funded. Apart from the mobility centres already mentioned, Whizz-Kidzs have set up special mobility centres for children, where expert advice is available (*www.whizz-kidz.org.uk*); this charity can also help with wheelchair funding.

People with Duchenne muscular dystrophy have complex wheelchair needs and it is still the case that the NHS wheelchair service struggles to provide good-quality wheelchairs for people with muscular dystrophy.

Referring people for wheelchair assessments is routine for occupational therapists. Occupational therapists can also be involved in the assessment and provision of wheelchairs. Wheelchair models change constantly and each NHS wheelchair service will provide different services. It is important to get up-to-date information on the wheelchairs that are available and what type of funding is obtainable before any assessments are carried out.

The Muscular Dystrophy Campaign can provide current detailed information on wheelchairs suitable for people with muscular dystrophy for occupational therapists who may not have experience of working with this client group. It is, however, still wise to try any chair before it is purchased (Muscular Dystrophy Campaign, 2006).

In the first instance, occupational therapists would normally refer a person with muscular dystrophy to the local NHS wheelchair service. Each of these services has its own criteria for provision, but they can normally fund or part-fund wheelchairs. Timescales from the date of referral to the actual provision of a wheelchair can be quite long. If the wheelchair service supplies a chair, find out who is responsible for maintaining the wheelchair and who is responsible for instructing the person on how to operate the wheelchair (Turner et al., 2002).

Transport is normally available to take you to the wheelchair centre where most assessments are conducted. It is advisable to take a professional worker along, such as a physiotherapist or an occupational therapist, who is familiar with the seating needs of the person with Duchenne muscular dystrophy and their family situation. They may be able to offer suggestions that will help to ensure that the seating provided meets the needs of the individual and the family.

Where the NHS wheelchair service has a problem funding the type of chair required by the individual, this can cause stress for all the family. It is often helpful for the family to have a social worker or another professional who can seek other funding sources for wheelchairs and other transport equipment. If the wheelchair is primarily needed for school purposes, the education department may fund the wheelchair, and, in some cases where the chair is needed to perform a range of functions in different areas, it may be the case that different functions of the chair may be funded by different agencies; a combination of NHS, social work and education funding may be used to secure the right chair for the individual.

When a wheelchair cannot be funded using these routes, there are many charities that can assist with funding, information and support. The value of the support that charities can offer to people with Duchenne muscular dystrophy should not be underestimated. They can provide good practical and financial support as well as a wealth of information and emotional support.

## INSURANCE

Cars and wheelchairs are valuable items; therefore, it is necessary for the owner to insure them to make certain that they can be replaced if they are damaged. Servicing agreements are also advisable for complex wheelchairs. Most companies will give quotes for servicing wheelchairs and cars prior to purchase. These costs can mount up, so it is an important factor to consider when selecting cars and wheelchairs.

## KEY POINTS

• Try wheelchairs and vehicles before purchasing.
• Make sure that the person, their wheelchair and their family can all access any proposed vehicle.
• Check the access available at every transfer stage of the journey.
• Apply for the benefits and grants that can help with transport costs.
• Check whether there are concessionary fares available.
• Make sure that the individual is positioned safely before starting a journey.

## CASE STUDY

The mother of a nine-year-old boy with Duchenne muscular dystrophy contacted her local social work occupational therapist, as she had difficulty parking her car near her home. The boy used a powered wheelchair for mobility and the family had a wheelchair-accessible vehicle on lease through the Motability scheme. The car was accessed via a ramp at the rear of the vehicle.

During a visit to the family home, the mother explained that she was often not able to park her car near her home due to the number of cars trying to park in the limited spaces available in the district. The house had no driveway or garage; therefore, it was agreed that the occupational therapist would request the provision of a disabled parking bay adjacent to the family home.

Normally, the occupational therapist would contact the local roads department to find out whether a parking bay could be provided on a specific road for a disabled person but, in this case, the house was located in a complex housing scheme, where the housing was located around a series of car parks. Therefore, the occupational therapist had to establish who actually owned the car park and then write to the owner to ask whether they would provide or give permission for a disabled parking bay to be marked out for this family.

The owner was a local housing association that refused the request, as the family had bought their home and they would not provide this service for people who were not tenants. The occupational therapist contacted the housing association again and asked for permission for a disabled parking bay to be painted for the family in the car park.

The housing association replied to the family and agreed that the family could have the parking bay if they paid for it to be painted at a cost of a few hundred pounds. The family reported this outcome to the occupational therapist and advised that they could not afford to pay for the parking bay to be painted. Following this, the occupational therapist again contacted the housing association to ask for permission to provide the parking bay at no cost to the housing association. The housing association eventually agreed.

In this case, the occupational therapist managed to get funding from social work to cover the cost of providing the disabled parking bay, as provision of the parking bay would assist the mother as a carer and reduce one stress on the family. The parking bay would also ensure that there was enough space at the rear of the car to allow the boy to access the car. Many times in the past, the rear access had been blocked by other cars parking too close.

The process of supplying the parking bay looks fairly straightforward, but the reality was that it took nearly two years from the original request for the disabled parking bay until it was finally provided. The delay points were getting decisions from the housing association, who felt that it was not an issue for them, as the request was not for one of their tenants, so it took a lot of pressure from local politicians before they would look at the request following their initial refusal.

Another delay was trying to identify who could legally paint the parking bay, as the roads department refused to paint the bay, as it was in a car park. The final delay was actually finding a dry day to paint the disabled parking bay.

## STUDY QUESTIONS

- Name three advantages of possessing a Blue Parking Badge.
- What is the safest position for a person travelling in a vehicle?
- What will the Hospital Travel Cost Scheme fund?
- What is a dangerous restraint for people travelling in their wheelchair?
- Who can travel free with a disabled person in a taxi?

# 16  Bereavement and Anticipatory Grief

## CLAIRE TESTER

## INTRODUCTION

As mentioned in Chapter 3, young men with Duchenne muscular dystrophy experience the loss of muscle strength, associated function and skills. The loss experienced is ongoing as the condition progresses. This loss is observed but not always understood by the health professional. In addition, as the young man reaches his late teens and early twenties, he becomes acutely aware of his own prognosis. This is compounded by the deterioration and death of his peers with Duchenne muscular dystrophy. These may be friendships formed through school, the Muscular Dystrophy Campaign, and/or the children's hospice. The impact of these deaths and the proximity to the young man himself cannot be underestimated, although it is not always fully recognised.

When a realisation or anxiety of impending loss is experienced in advance of the loss, this is anticipatory loss (Tester, 2007). Anticipatory loss can be experienced by people close to the person, too. This will be discussed after bereavement.

Some of the processes of anticipatory bereavement and of bereavement and loss will be discussed here to provide an insight for the therapist in order to inform the therapeutic approach.

## LOSS

Loss is understood as a want (for someone or something missing), an injury and defeat, as in lost (Longman, 1976). It is also used to describe bereavement. To lose something also involves seeking to find or recover the lost object. There is a period of missing what has been lost, involving pining or want. This period is replaced by an acceptance of having lost, and the re-adjustment to living without what has been lost. Thinking about the loss of muscle power and of movement in Duchenne muscular dystrophy, it is cumulative and progressive. Presently, there is no way that these losses can be prevented and the person experiencing these losses of strength of their own being is powerless in the face of this progression. One's own physical abilities are usually taken for granted and not considered, but thought needs to be given to the experience of the loss of muscle power for boys and young men.

In Duchenne muscular dystrophy, paralysis is gradual and creeping. To consider the emotional response to this loss, or losses, it is necessary to understand some of the behavioural patterns which can occur and inform the therapeutic management and approach. The loss of one's own muscle strength, function and skills can be compared to bereavement of aspects of one's self. In this way, the process of mourning, which is perceived as normal, although profoundly emotionally distressing, can occur for the young person with Duchenne muscular dystrophy. Therapists working with boys with Duchenne muscular dystrophy and their families may present as accepting and unsurprised, even blasé, by the new loss of function that a child presents with. This attitude can be disturbing for the child and parent. It is always helpful to begin by asking the boy how he is managing and whether there are any things that he is having difficulty with. In this way, the therapist becomes part of helping to recover the loss by looking at how to help with function through positioning, assessment and provision of aids, including technology, where necessary. It is first important to acknowledge with the boy and his family their *own* experience of loss rather than to project the therapist's own perceptions and belief upon the family. It is necessary to always start where the young person is, and this involves listening first.


## BEREAVEMENT

Bereavement is acknowledged as a normal process after the death of someone close. However, the encompassing and profound grief affects the person's ability to cope with normal day-to-day activities. This is recognised in society – compassionate leave is given by a workplace in recognition of the need for the person to have time to come to terms with their grief, and acknowledging difficulties in carrying on with regular tasks. There are different theoretical models of bereavement which view the mourning process as variantly having tasks, stages, emotional states, a set of strategies and behaviours. The length of time required to recover or readjust to the loss of the person cannot be determined, as it is personal and unique to everyone.

Freud identified that the more profound the loss to the individual, the greater the impact and the longer it takes to accept the loss, if at all (Freud, 1917). He also recognised that mourning as seen in bereavement can be experienced as not only the loss or death of a person, but as the loss of an ideal, liberty or an abstract concept linked to the self. This could include the sense of one's future self, such as the realisation of oneself as a future paralysed self rather than a physically active person.

Bereavement has been viewed as something one recovers from (Guntripp, 1992); this view encourages the idea that something is left behind and forgotten in order to move on. This is a linear view which Murray Parkes (1998) identified as having four main stages, beginning with disbelief, active searching and anger, moving to despair, followed by adjustment and acceptance. This appears to echo a medical model of process and recovery (Greenstreet, 2004) but, whilst these stages can be identified, they are not clear-cut and do not always follow this order. Walter (1996) proposed a bereavement process which required a biography of the loss – of finding a sense and meaning in it. This loss is reabsorbed emotionally, with reference to what or who is no longer present and remembered. Walter maintained that whatever has been lost has been, and continues to be, part of the emotional being of the person experiencing the bereavement and cannot be forgotten or left behind.

Stroebe and Schut (1999) proposed a different model, recognising that a person may move backwards and forwards through different tasks of coping with bereavement. They defined these tasks or activities as being either loss-oriented or restoration-oriented. These tasks could include the organising of the funeral of the deceased whilst still being in an emotional state of disbelief. For someone who has lost muscle function, unable to stand and walk independently, this could involve the active use of a wheelchair, whilst still wanting to stand and walk. Stroebe and Schut (1999) recognised that a person is not emotionally static but moves between different states of appearing to cope, whilst unable to adjust and accept what has occurred. This dynamic model shows no set pattern, recognising that the pace and the process are defined by the individual and that it is a unique experience. This raises a question of what is not a normal bereavement. How can someone be recognised as having difficulties in grieving or being 'stuck' in bereavement? Whilst this cannot be fully addressed here, it is essentially when a person presents with *ongoing* problems in daily functioning affecting their own health and well-being, or that of others, which needs to be recognised as requiring referral to mental health services.

Bereavement can be understood to be an emotional and psychological event, which may occur several times in one's life. It affects one's sense of well-being and provokes questions of a spiritual and religious nature, challenging one's existence, sense of meaning and purpose. Bereavement and the associated mourning can also accompany traumatic loss of aspects of oneself, as in paralysis, injury and relationship breakdown. Thought needs to be given to the fragility of one's confidence, self-esteem and identity when a young person is still growing and developing with a deteriorating condition. It is not always recognised that children grieve, as bereavement is often understood to belong to adulthood.

## ANTICIPATORY GRIEF

Anticipatory grief or anticipatory bereavement can be experienced for some time before the event of a loss. It is in anticipation of something which is expected or understood will happen and this loss is actively worked through as a bereavement process, even when the person or object of anticipated loss is present. This means that a person can 'work' through aspects of mourning because of the *anticipated* loss, not through a specific event. When an event occurs, this anticipatory loss does not assuage the bereavement process; it is still potent and occurs (Corr et al., 1997). Anticipatory grief can involve a heightened concern for the person or object which is feared will be lost, and a rehearsal or practice of the loss played out in the mind of the person, with considerations of readjustments to the loss (Tester, 2007). This can occur for some parents when they are given the prognosis for Duchenne muscular dystrophy when their children are infants or small boys. This may also occur for the young men themselves. The emotional pain that this entails is considerable and seldom acknowledged formally. Young men may become aware of the feelings and emotions of close relatives and this can compound the difficulty of keeping up cheerful appearances for the benefit of parents. As hospice staff have remarked (see Chapter 17), such thoughts of loss and anticipated grief are present but held within by these young men. Anticipatory grief creates a tension which is privately held, and inadvertently causes a waiting.


## WHEN SOMEONE DIES

As mentioned earlier, young men with Duchenne muscular dystrophy may encounter bereavement from the death of peers with the same condition. Sometimes, these deaths may be of relatives or close friends. As one mother described:

> 'He has "lost" four friends with DMD now and has become very withdrawn and although I want to protect him from knowing about these deaths, I cannot as he is in regular email contact with his friends. He has become very philosophical now, but his mood is heavy, as he asks – Will I be next?'

As seen, bereavement is a normal process and is experienced by young men with Duchenne muscular dystrophy; it may be heightened with the knowledge of their own condition, but not necessarily. It needs to be recognised and the person helped to work through the process of grief. For some, this can involve writing a piece, like a biography, in remembering the friendship of the person; for others, help from a priest or chaplain in offering and remembrance can be helpful. Attending the funeral or visiting the grave of the person to say goodbye is helpful in the bereavement process, but not always offered due to the protection and sensitivities of the parents of a son with Duchenne muscular dystrophy, or those of the health professionals involved. It should be remembered that when a young person is experiencing bereavement, then melancholy thoughts and feelings which they may share with the health professional can involve thoughts of their own sense of self, which is both normal in bereavement and particularly acute.

Parents of the young man may also be more acutely affected by the death of their son's friend with Duchenne muscular dystrophy and this should be acknowledged.

## IN SUMMARY

Loss and anticipatory bereavement are not confined to working with Duchenne muscular dystrophy, as these aspects cut across other physical and mental health conditions which the occupational therapist encounters. However, it is necessary to be both aware and sensitive to the possibility of the different experiences and depths of loss when working with children and young people with Duchenne muscular dystrophy. The focus at all times for the occupational therapist is on living and enabling independence but the attitude and approach of the therapist are fundamental to a positive working relationship with the young man and his family. Unfortunately, due to the key role of the occupational therapist, there have been occasions on which a family has been upset by the therapist's manner. This helps no one and is unnecessary. Tact, sensitivity and diplomacy are required by the occupational therapist together with an insight into the difficulties which a family may be experiencing.

## KEY POINTS

- Bereavement can be experienced by a person of their future self, or of skills or muscle power.
- Loss and bereavement affect a person emotionally, psychologically and physically.
- Anticipatory grief or loss can occur for some time before an anticipated event.
- It is necessary to consider aspects of loss, in a sensitive therapeutic approach.
- Bereavement support may be needed for the young man with Duchenne muscular dystrophy, and for the family when a friend dies.

## CASE STUDY

Ian is a young man of 18 years. He lives at home with his parents. He has just left school, and does not have any plans at present. He has just taken possession of a new powered wheelchair – a tilt-in-space chair, as Ian can no longer adjust his own sitting position to relieve pressure. His parents notice that he is unusually flat in his mood. This has been for two weeks now and he is reluctant to go out. His parents are concerned that it is because of any uncertainty about the new wheelchair. As he has left school, he no longer sees the school physiotherapist for his passive exercises, nor does he see his occupational therapist. Many of his friends from school (mainstream) are preparing to go on to university or college and to live away from home.

- What might be contributing to Ian's 'flat' mood?
- How might he be supported? And by whom?

## STUDY QUESTIONS

- Choose two theories of bereavement and, exploring them further, discuss the differences and similarities.
- Explain bereavement, grief and anticipatory loss/grief.
- Consider the experience of losing muscle strength, and associated skills and abilities, and how this might affect adolescence.
- Discuss the statement that 'Bereavement is a normal process'.

# 17 The Role of the Hospice

CLAIRE TESTER

## INTRODUCTION

Many boys and young adults with Duchenne muscular dystrophy are known to children's hospices, but not all. As not all boys with Duchenne muscular dystrophy are referred to a children's hospice, or their parents or health professionals do not consider the hospice as having a part to play, it raises the question of what is the function of the children's hospice in Duchenne muscular dystrophy. Thinking about the role of the children's hospices, it would be helpful to define what a hospice is, the difference between children's hospices and adults' hospices, and also to define palliative care before discussing what is being provided for families and their sons with Duchenne muscular dystrophy.

## HOSPICES AND PALLIATIVE CARE

A hospice originated as a place of refuge, or rest, provided by a monastic order for weary travellers on pilgrimages. It has now defined as a programme, or a facility, to provide palliative care and attend to emotional, physical, spiritual and social needs of terminally ill patients and their families, at the hospice or within the home (Dorlands, 2005). The emphasis is on the relief of pain and promoting quality of life. In this way, it can be seen that hospice care has developed into a concept of care, as it is not limited to the hospice building itself.

The hospice movement was pioneered by Dame Cicely Saunders in London in the 1960s, in recognition of the pain and palliative care needs of people with terminal cancer. Voluntary organisations such as Marie Curie developed hospices for cancer patients. People with non-malignant conditions were recognised as having palliative care needs and further hospices were established. All of these hospices were for adults with terminal conditions to provide end-of-life care, and a supportive environment in which to die. In 1981, the first children's hospice in the world was opened for children at Helen House,

Oxford. This was for children with life-limiting conditions and palliative care needs for malignant and non-malignant conditions, providing respite for the whole family, short stays and support, as well as terminal care for the child when required.

There are more children's hospices in the UK and around the world which use this original model of palliative care support for the child and family, providing respite care, as well as end-of-life care. Support also includes bereavement support for the family after the death of a child or young person, too.

Palliative care has become recognised as a specific field of medical practice (Hynson & Sawyer, 2001). Palliative care was originally understood as providing terminal care for a person at the end of life, but this has been developed to provide care for non-curative and life-limiting conditions. As children may be diagnosed with life-limiting conditions, such as Duchenne muscular dystrophy, at birth or in the early years, it can be argued that these children and their families are regarded as having palliative care needs. The World Health Organisation defines palliative care for children as including 'the care of the child's body, mind and spirit' as well as support to the family. The goal of palliative care is achievement of the best quality of life for patients and families (WHO, 1998). However, whilst palliative care implies 'doing for' the person, and caring for them, it does also involve working *with* the person to address all of their needs to 'work towards the best quality of life which is both unique and personal to each person' (Tester, 2007). This involves supporting and developing the potential of the person to be as independent as possible, which involves making decisions and choices for oneself, being as active as possible and living life to the full.

The term 'palliative rehabilitation' has been developed in recognition that there is an ongoing adaptation and a re-adjustment to living with a deteriorating condition (Bray & Cooper, 2003). Thinking about children, it needs to be recognised that they are growing and developing, learning about the world around them and needing to explore and engage with it. Children's needs in palliative care are very different from adult palliative care needs, and children's hospices reflect this. A children's hospice provides support to the growing child and the whole family, including siblings and grandparents. The multidisciplinary team often includes nurses, a Physiotherapist, an Occupational Therapist, a Social Worker, a Youth Worker, a Chaplain and care workers, including volunteers and complementary health therapists.

A children's hospice may provide support to a family over several years, according to the family's needs, which may not involve a respite stay for some time. So where do boys and young men with Duchenne muscular dystrophy fit in with hospice care? Are they in need of palliative care, or rather palliative rehabilitation? As has been shown, the understanding of hospice care has changed and continues to evolve, as does palliative care. Hospices are still associated with death and dying for many, whilst the emphasis of children's hospices includes making the most of life and living, providing support where needed. In addition, the prognosis of Duchenne muscular dystrophy is changing as medical advances are made and, significantly, overnight ventilation has extended life into the twenties, thirties and, for some individuals, into the forties. There are also boys who have Duchenne muscular dystrophy who do not use overnight ventilation, and may have a fast deteriorating condition. Already, it can be seen that there are differences in needs.

## ROLE OF THE HOSPICE

So, in considering the role of the children's hospice, it was necessary to ask some of the children's hospices about the services provided to boys and young men with Duchenne muscular dystrophy. Presently, boys with Duchenne muscular dystrophy may be known to a hospice but are not referred until they are using a powered wheelchair and have identified needs for support. For some hospices, this is around 16 years of age. This support may be defined as respite for the family and the boy, or as support which may be in recognition of social needs. Respite care may be a weekend or overnight stay to give the parents a break, or even the boy a break from his family in order to spend time with other boys at the hospice with the same condition.

Hospice staff have recognised that boys with Duchenne muscular dystrophy can be isolated and do not come into contact with other boys with the same condition unless they are in the same family. Consequently, some children's hospices have developed teenage weekends specifically to address the social needs of the boys. As adolescence has markedly different stages (see Chapter 13), these teenage weekends have been developed for younger teens and for older teens or, rather, young adults. The younger teen weekends have been devised with the intention of fun and normality as much as possible. This includes going out to the cinema, visiting McDonalds on the way, late nights and opportunities to chat and share in activities centred on sport and other shared interests. These occasions have enabled these adolescents to meet and enjoy the company of others with the same condition, and to experience being a member of a group, and sharing experiences. In turn, the sharing of contact details has led to friendships being continued after these times through email and phone contact.

Staff recognise that this peer support is an important aspect of these weekends, and also helps to build a relationship with staff over time. This relationship is ongoing and as it involves personal care such as bathing, toileting, dressing and help with preparing food to eat, the adolescents experience at first hand the care and attention provided by staff. This leads to a trust in the relationship, and opportunities for discussing any concerns and questions which can be put to staff for honest and open discussion on a one-to-one basis. These include topics which might not be addressed with parents.

The weekends for older teens or, rather, young adults are planned actively with them. This has included requested talks and discussions on the affects of alcohol and smoking, about sex and of specific concerns which arise. As the hospice has a duty of care and is in a position of loco parentis, nothing is encouraged which would be harmful or unsuitable. For example, if further information is required by an individual, such as sexual counselling, then information or contact details may be given if a member of staff considers this appropriate, after a one-to-one discussion with the person. Whilst children's hospices also provide support to parents and siblings, the teen weekends have been exclusively for the adolescents with the hospice 'taken over' by them so that they might be encouraged to enjoy a sense of freedom and independence. Activities have involved outings to major sports events and, where age-appropriate, to a pub and to concerts. Events which might normally be too difficult to access without parental help but which might be difficult to do with them, such as attending a heavy rock concert, are possible with the support of the children's hospice and, in addition, they have others with the same interest and condition to accompany them. This is living life, and being enabled to partake in it, and to enjoy it.

Some of the activities that a children's hospice organises may be surprising, as they involve risk, but the emphasis is on building the self-confidence of the young person, and an introduction to a new view of what is possible which they may never have considered before. Some of these activities include outward-bound trips involving staying over at a hostel and participating fully in abseiling, archery, zip-wiring, sailing and motor-boating. These activities are all adapted for wheelchairs and with specially trained instructors. These trips can involve meeting others all staying at the same lodge and from different areas, leading to opportunities to form new relationships and to compete with them, too. Staff assess who is able to go on these trips, regarding the young person's health and also from a safety point of view. The benefits are always positive. As one young man said of abseiling, 'I thought, I cannot do that, go up in the air, I just can't. But I did! It felt so good. I have photos to prove it. My mum said she would have been so worried if she had been there and knew what I was doing, but she wasn't!'

This is another aspect of taking part in new activities and being away from home, as the young men have an opportunity to experience life out of the home, and without their parents. Some children's hospices also encourage opportunities to meet and take part in activities with able-bodied peers, involving local community groups and organisations such as the Scout movement. One venture involved camping near to the hospice and being outdoors for the whole weekend. The experience was regarded as very positive by both groups of young men and opened up a different view for both. Befriender schemes overseen by youth workers at a hospice encourage socialising with peers, within and outwith the hospice.

Whilst involving the young men with their able-bodied peers in appropriate activities, there is also the recognition that these young men also need to get together as a group to discuss shared concerns. These are addressed in discussion groups at which questions of how the condition progresses and options in medical management are also raised at these weekends – questions such as 'What will happen to me when I get unwell?' Information and demonstrations have included using urine sheaths, spinal fusion, overnight ventilation and the different model options, such as nasal prongs or over-mouth mask, naso–gastric tube feeding and gastrostomy, and tracheostomy. Some hospices provide this information in-house, whilst others encourage medical or community staff to be invited for a specific discussion issue. Hospice staff have been surprised at how discussions are readily initiated by these young men on the deterioration of health and of the need to share thinking on the different interventions available to them and of their own preferences. This has led to end-of-life care planning for some young men, who have often already considered what they would like, or not like and seeking an opportunity to discuss this on a one-to-one basis with a member of staff, and for it to be documented. This often involves the youth worker, who has the most contact, but not always. As one member of staff remarked, 'He was so keen to discuss it all, and said he had been thinking about this for some time but did not wish to upset his parents by bringing it all out in the open. With time and encouragement we did involve his mother in the discussion, and afterwards she said she was so relieved as she did not know what he wanted, but didn't know how to discuss it.'

As children's hospices provide end-of-life care, and care of the body after death for a few days, there is usually a bedroom set aside, which is part of the hospice building but apart from the other bedrooms. During the end-of-life discussions initiated by the young men in the older teenage weekends, there have been requests to view the room, and comments made on how they would like the room to be when they might use it after their own death. Whilst this is a difficult subject both to contemplate and to discuss, the hospice staff have recognised that these thoughts are held by these young men who have real difficulty discussing them with their family, and these requests are initiated always by the young men themselves: 'In a way, because it has already been talked about, and my wishes are known, then I don't have to worry about it anymore and can just get on with living life,' said one man of 20 years with Duchenne muscular dystrophy.

Such discussions also raise the question of where the young man wishes to be and of the interventions he wants, which he may not be able to influence at the critical stage. An individual's preferences have ranged from no intervention, and to be taken to the children's hospice for end-of-life care or after death, to requesting acute intervention of cardiac resuscitation and tracheostomy. It should be stressed that this end-of-life care planning is discussed with young men who are of adult status, but they are encouraged and supported to share their plans with their parents. On occasion, staff have been requested to act as advocates in having the discussion with the parents with the young man present, or nearby, when it is too emotionally difficult for the son to broach the subject with his parents.

Staff see relationships develop over time between the young men themselves and also with the staff. In this way, the hospice is seen as a safe environment in which discussions and sharing of thoughts, feelings and concerns can be brought. This building of relationships and respect for the individual are at the core of the role of the children's hospice. As one member of staff put it, 'We are also making good memories too, having good times together'. The weekend events and activities, although they are planned and coordinated in advance, encourage active participation, with as much spontaneous fun and enjoyment as is possible. Whilst there are serious times, the emphasis is on enjoying one's youth and being encouraged to be as independent as possible.

As this level of support and palliative rehabilitation is not matched by other existing services, young men with Duchenne muscular dystrophy do acknowledge the unique support that the hospice can provide. However, as they move into their twenties, there is a recognition by some of them that they have outgrown a children's hospice. The difficulty is that adult hospices do not provide this level of service and support, and, unfortunately, the young men can become isolated. This raises the question of where and by whom the needs of these young men can be met, and of the transition of services from children to adult services. Parents are also caught up in this difficulty, as they may have developed relationships with staff at a children's hospice over years, and have difficulty in ending this trust and familiarity when there isn't an equivalent service to move on to.

It is questioned whether a children's hospice is an appropriate referral in the first place at all, as it can introduce the possibility of dying to a young adolescent who may not have been considered before. Often, children's hospices do request that parents inform a child about the nature of a hospice before their first visit. This is interpreted by different parents in different ways, and has included explanations of a hospice; as a hotel, a place for a holiday and an extension of a hospital. This may also reflect the difficulty that a parent has in both accepting a hospice as well as describing it to their son. Some parents have said that if they were to explain what a hospice is, this would include the fact that some children may be there because they are dying. This is too painful for a parent to acknowledge, and might lead to their own son's asking more about his own condition which has not been discussed with the parent. As shown, hospices provide much more than terminal care, and Duchenne muscular dystrophy, too, has an extended prognosis, but still there is a real difficulty in parents' sharing both what they understand and know about the condition, and relaying it to their son. This reluctance on the part of the parent has led to some confusion and anxiety for boys and young men staying at the hospice for the first time. The confusion and anxiety have been due to encountering other children who are physically unwell and with other conditions who also have profound developmental delay; of sometimes being amongst much younger children, which had been off-putting; and, occasionally, because a child at the hospice had been very unwell and in their terminal stage of care, which the boy with Duchenne muscular dystrophy became aware of. In addition, an initial stay at the hospice may not have involved the parent(s) staying over as well, depending upon family circumstances, and this has caused an unease and anxiety for the boy.

When talking to parents about the difficulty in discussing a hospice with their son(s), and considering the service that a hospice can provide, it was evident that the initial suggestion of being referred to a hospice had been distressing, as a hospice had been associated with death and dying. Whereas, for the parents who had been introduced to the idea of a hospice, had met with hospice staff before visiting the hospice and then had the visit itself, they had all been pleasantly surprised by how different it was in reality from their own image and perception of how it might be. By contrast, parents who refused to accept a referral to a hospice for their son for respite or home support were adamant that their son was not going to die before reaching adulthood, and that involvement with a hospice was supporting a view which was reinforcing a life-limiting condition which could remove a sense of hope and future for their son. This last view is worth exploring, as it raises more questions about the role of the hospice and the understanding of Duchenne muscular dystrophy. Does association with a children's hospice reinforce a negative view of one's own life as being limited and affect one's own perception of a limited future, with morbid thoughts?

Often, at children's hospices there are photographs and/or names of children who have died at the hospice, and who are actively remembered. These details are usually in a prominent place and unintentionally reinforce that the hospice is for children who are dying and die. This can be distressing for the parents as well as unsettling for the young men with Duchenne muscular dystrophy. This aspect might reinforce a sense of fatalism. As one 17-year-old at a children's hospice commented, 'I take a day at a time. That's all I can do'. This comment indicates a sense of resignation and of almost defeatism that planning into the future was difficult and perhaps impossible. This view was reinforced by his own family, who had been given the limited prognosis *as it used to be*, when he was an infant, that he would die in his mid-teens. It is difficult to say whether the negative view of this young man and his future is exacerbated by the hospice or in fact provides him with activity and social contact that he would not otherwise receive at home. In contrast, other young adults use the children's hospice services as a resource in helping where appropriate, in realising their social activities and future plans. As one mother commented on her 18-year-old son with Duchenne muscular dystrophy, 'He's never in. He's always out. And when he needs help to do something he's on the phone to the Youth worker at the hospice to get the information'. Some young men take the initiative themselves in recognising how they wish to use the hospice, preferring not to use the facility itself, but the service itself as an outreach. For families having a relationship with hospice staff, knowing that they are there can be reassuring for when they may need it. As one doctor commented, 'Sometimes young men with DMD can deteriorate quickly, and the family want to use the hospice for care and support. Also sometimes a young man may die suddenly from an acute pulmonary event'. The hospice offers an opportunity to optimise medical care and support, liaising with medical and nursing colleagues, and reviewing needs where necessary. For example, when a young man has a chest infection, a parent may request a stay at the hospice for care, including medical and physiotherapy input.

## SUMMARY

The role of the hospice would appear to be both complex and flexible at the same time. It essentially comes down to the individual boy and his family in their understanding of the condition, the understanding of the role of the children's hospice, which is different from an adult hospice, and what services are being received presently to address the young man's needs for rehabilitation and social activity. As one mother remarked, 'I want my son to be sociable and active in his own community and that means getting involved with children his own age. Just because he is the only one in a wheelchair and with DMD doesn't mean he shouldn't be there (at the hospice). And it doesn't mean he should be in a ghetto of other boys with DMD either'.

Sometimes, as a boy grows older and his condition progresses, his need for social inclusion changes, as does the parents' need for support. These are personal decisions and reflect the need for regarding everyone as unique and individual, with needs which can fluctuate at different times, which includes individual members within the same family. As one father admitted, 'My son and my wife came here (children's hospice) and I never wanted any part in it. I wouldn't even come to the door. I thought the idea of a children's hospice was all wrong. We used to argue about it, my wife and I. She said it helped her though. Now I am here on a Family Fun day, I can see what it does. It is not how I imagined it to be'.

In recognition of the changing needs of young adults who have a life-limiting condition but, due to medical advances, are living well and longer, the children's hospice, Helen House, has opened a respite home called Douglas House, describing it as a 'Respite service' for people aged between 16 and 40 years. The emphasis is still on support and palliative care, including end-of-life care, but social needs are recognised, with a cinema and a bar. This could be the future step for children's hospices as medical advances enable young adults with life-limiting conditions to live longer. The need for respite for themselves and for their families, with the opportunity to socialise with others and to develop palliative rehabilitation with opportunities to live independently, may be part of the provision of children's hospice services, with government funding in the future. The opportunity to live independently in community housing away from the hospice for short stays with staff is also a possible future service by a hospice. As ongoing medical advances are made in Duchenne muscular dystrophy, the role of the hospice is challenged.

## KEY POINTS

• A hospice provides palliative care *and* end-of-life care.
• A children's hospice is different from an adult hospice.
• A children's hospice provides support to the child, young adult and the family, too.
• The palliative care provided by a children's hospice is flexible to suit the needs of the individual.
• Not everyone with Duchenne muscular dystrophy needs to be referred to a hospice.
• A children's hospice can meet needs not met by any existing services.

## CASE STUDY

Neil has been known to the children's hospice for five years, since he was 15. He uses the hospice for respite, and his parents have got to know other parents whose sons have Duchenne muscular dystrophy. They meet up, even when not at the hospice. Neil has enjoyed the activity weekends which are held during the year, and has also been able to attend a concert of his favourite band with hospice staff support. He knows the staff well. However, he is moving house due to his Dad's new job. He will not be able to attend the hospice, as he will be out of the catchment area. Neil is quite worried about all the change and upheaval that he is to face. The hospice staff, with his permission, find out about services available to him in his new area. They also promise to visit him. The Youth Worker finds out about activities and groups in his area, and the Social Worker, Physiotherapist and Occupational Therapist provide contact names and addresses of their counterparts in Neil's new area for his information. There is not a children's hospice in the new area, but there is an adult hospice. Neither Neil nor his parents wishes to link with this hospice yet.

Consider why Neil will miss the children's hospice but does not wish to link with the adult hospice.

## STUDY QUESTIONS

- What do you understand as the key points that a hospice can provide?
- What are the positive aspects of referring a young man and his family?

# 18 In Conversation with Occupational Therapists

CLAIRE TESTER

## INTRODUCTION

Occupational Therapists may be involved with the same child and family over years or for a one-off specific referral request. Sometimes, despite the best intentions and a sensitive approach, intervention does not always go according to plan. This can be both upsetting and frustrating for the therapist in meeting their duty of care. For the majority of Occupational Therapists, intervention goes well, and good working relationships are made with the family and other health professionals. In conversation with different occupational therapists, the view is that when something does not go well or smoothly, it can be felt as a failure by the therapist. This provides opportunities for reflection. Each of the comments shared below have been given by different therapists, to provide an insight and to inform learning. Thanks are given to the honesty of the therapists in acknowledging and sharing their experiences:

'I received a referral from the Paediatrician for an 8 year old boy with DMD with regard to an assessment of a manual wheelchair. I contacted the Physiotherapist at the school who was working with the child, and it was agreed that I would arrange to visit the parents first. However what I did not realise was that no one has raised the possibility of a wheelchair in the near future. Also too that when I went to visit the mother at home that the family lived in a first floor flat. The mother was very angry that I should be suggesting a wheelchair. She said that the Physiotherapist was maintaining her son's walking and standing, and that I was going to jeopardise this. It was very difficult too in asking if she had considered moving home to a ground floor flat. All round, the mother seemed to think I was both interfering and negative.

Afterwards I wished I had suggested that either the Physio or the Paediatrician introduced me to the parent after discussing the indications for a manual wheelchair for her son. I think too there was a need for someone to spend time with the parents on what was understood by Duchenne muscular dystrophy and how this would affect the family accommodation. As it was I had to go back to the Physiotherapist and the Paediatrician and tell them what had happened. A meeting was held at the school with the teaching staff, the Physiotherapist, and myself to identify the best way to approach the situation. The parents were then invited into school by the teacher and Physio, and they raised the need for a wheelchair with the parents. They explained it would be helpful for their son to have to hand when the boy was tired, or on school outings. The Physio then involved me. The accommodation issue has not been broached properly in my view, but if there was to be a fire in the building the lifts would be out of action and the boy would have to be carried down. I am meeting the Paediatrician and Physiotherapist this week to discuss future accommodation needs, and how we can, as a team, introduce this. I am also seeing the Family Care Officer from the Muscular Dystrophy Campaign who is working with the family.'

'Addressing needs in the home can be difficult. There seem to be constant changes the parents have to accept in their son as he loses skills and abilities which is distressing, and then to compound or it seems to reinforce the increasing dependence and disability of their son, the O.T. suggests equipment and changes in the home. Sometimes you can see the real difference a piece of equipment would make to the family, yet they resist it. I can think of one family I was visiting and the mother had a really bad backache. Her son needed to transfer and I looked around for the portable hoist so that I could help. I asked where it was, and the mum got a bit embarrassed. She said it was in the garage. She said she had never used it. She and her husband wanted to lift their son for all transfers. When I asked her gently on a 1:1 if this was perhaps how she had hurt her back, she said she wanted to hold her son, as it was quicker, and that she felt it would be treating her son as a 'load' she couldn't manage if she were to use the hoist. It was a shame as her son felt guilty that his mother's back problem was caused by him.'

'Although a family has a hoist supplied, it is surprising that parents prefer to lift manually. On one home visit, the mother told me not to speak or move, as she lifted her son and carried him from his wheelchair to the bed. Although her son was of a slight build she had to almost fold his legs up as she lifted him, but as he landed on the bed, he fell to the side. There was nothing dignified about it. Fortunately the young man did not have a spinal fusion, as she would not have been able to do this. It was very difficult being put in a position of watching this. Afterwards I said to her quietly that whilst I respected it was her home, her son did not look very comfortable, and too that he was growing all of the time. When was she going to consider introducing a hoist? It did lead to a further discussion about moving and handling safely. I did get to reassure her that I was there to provide support and advice to help, not to act as some form of moving and handling policing.'

'Hoists and transfers seem to be a difficult issue. One father was rude to me when I was suggesting a hoist for the home, and told me that he was physically strong enough and capable of carrying his son. He seemed to think it was unmanly to use a hoist or any transfer equipment. I managed to introduce the idea of a hoist as being necessary to the carers who were just starting to visit the home to get the young man ready for school.'

'Thinking about hoists, there is an upheaval in the home when an overhead hoist is installed. Although these can be preferable because they are less obtrusive than a large standing hoist, there needs to be a ceiling supporting beam. This can inter-fere with doorways, and lighting fittings. Sometimes families do not want all of this marking of the ceilings and walls. It is difficult to answer the question, How will I sell this house when I need to? It really is a choice the family make. As an O.T. I can only advise.'

A Social Services Occupational Therapist was in discussions with the family for adaptations and of the ongoing needs of the son. There was a difficulty when the mother refused to agree to the changes, as she insisted that an exten-sion to the house was necessary, not a reorganisation within the house. This led to an impasse, as the parent accused the Social Services Occupational Therapist as misrepresenting her. The Occupational Therapist remarks:

'It was very difficult as I had to work within the budget. I had to identify the most reasonable option in light of monies and needs. The parents seemed to feel that I was being mean, and not even-handed. It came to light that a family they knew had had an extension paid for by Social Services. This family was in another area and had access to a different fund of monies, and too his needs were different. It became very difficult to work with the family as I tried to explain the position and what they were eligible for. They made a complaint against me and refused to see me. They requested another O.T.. I felt such a failure, and my confidence fell to an all time low. The other O.T. said the same as me. The parents decided to raise money for an extension to their house. The equipment needed was reviewed in light of this. I did not work with the family again. I felt like a scapegoat really for the difficulties the family were having.'

'When I was working in community paediatrics a young boy was referred for Occupational Therapy re. seating. He enjoyed his school which was small, and he knew everyone, and they knew him. He saw his Physiotherapist weekly and we worked together on transfers, and on the introduction of a manual wheelchair when needed. This was a good working relationship. However when the time came for him to move to secondary school he was very reluctant to visit it in his last summer term at primary school. As therapists we went and checked access and the suitability of the environment. We linked with both parents and teaching staff too. But when the new term began he refused to go to school. His mum suggested that we meet him at the school at the beginning of term as she took him in. But what we did not recognise was that this boy seemed to think it was all a conspiracy against him and the physio and myself were engineering this change. He refused to speak to us, to actively partake in any therapy at all. He showed real hate in his eyes and no matter how much we explained to him, he would stare at us, and then turn away. He extended this silence to the teaching staff too. We discussed this with the teaching staff, and with the parents. We suggested a change in thera-pists. This did occur for a few sessions, but the parents asked for us to carry on as before. They said we were the connection with the primary school. But the young man still refuses to speak to us. It is wearing. It has gone on for a year now and I suppose we kept thinking he cannot keep this going, but somehow it has become permanent and we all work round it with message board, and hand signs to indicate needs. It is time for some intervention from a psychologist.'

'Having worked with a young man and his family for several years now I can feel my concern and worry as he gets older. I think I have become too close to the family, and feel it might be time to involve another therapist in the department.'

*'Are you worried in some way of becoming over involved?'*

'Yes. I don't think I would be able to cope with my work with this family or any other if the young man becomes ill. But I don't want to let the mother down. She and I have a good working relationship. She says I am a good support for her.'

*'Have you discussed this with your manager? It might be possible to share this work with another therapist so that it doesn't feel as if it all falling to you. If there was some acknowledged support within your department this might help you. It may not be necessary to have an all or nothing relationship with the family.'*

'I had not considered that. It would be a good idea.'

'A young man I am involved with for his powered wheelchair has become house bound it seems. He has left school and does not have any plans for attending higher education. He stays at home with his mother, who does not drive. When I see him he appears more physically frail. His mother says that he prefers to lie on his bed in a semi-reclined position, away from the family. His mother has become concerned about his eating as he eats very slowly and seems to lose interest in food, and does not show much interest in anything else.

I suggested that perhaps he was depressed and needed to see a doctor. She disagreed. It is a very difficult situation. There is no father around, nor any siblings. They only have each other. I have been providing regular feedback to the Consultant Neurologist. The Physiotherapist is not permitted into the house as his mother says that physical exercise will tire him. I was hoping that she could provide an assessment. The Consultant has suggested an urgent review with mother and son, as both would attend this meeting with him. This is now set for next week, but I am concerned that the young man is so weak he will have difficulty attending the hospital. I am very worried that this young man is depressed, and is starving himself. I am still able to visit the home, but I feel very isolated. I have kept my manager up to date on this. What is hard is that the young man is an adult and able to make his own choices which involves refusing treatment and intervention. The Consultant Neurologist has suggested a total review and assessment with a short admission to hospital.

In retrospect I think he lost so much when he left school, he didn't keep up with his friends, and he seemed somehow to have lost hope too. I think his mum still had the view of the 'old' prognosis of dying in middle teens. Somehow they seem as if they are waiting, rather than living.'

'In contrast a young man I have been working with has completed his degree at university and had a lot of support from the university and from the local services. He has a degree in IT and has gone on to do some freelance work. He is presently considering living independently, and already employs his own carers whom he also interviewed himself. He is a very independently minded person and has travelled abroad with his carers on holiday. It has taken planning, but he has done it. He always challenges me to problem solve, and sometimes he finds information on equipment and services I don't know about, which he finds on the internet.'

## KEY POINTS

* The therapeutic relationship with the parents and the boy or young adult is important, and the approach needs to be thought of right at the start.
* Things don't always go smoothly; we are all human and can make mistakes.
* There is a need for helpful reflection to gain insight into what you have done, and how you might improve a situation.

## STUDY QUESTIONS

* From these comments, the importance of the relationship with the parents in the early years and the relationship with the young man is apparent. Choose one of these scenarios above and, in light of building good relationships, consider your approach.
* From one of the above scenarios, consider the effect of the situation upon (a) the young man; (b) the parents; and (c) the therapist.

# 19 The Future

CLAIRE TESTER AND DR ALISON WILCOX

Duchenne muscular dystrophy is an inherited X-linked recessive condition (although, in a third of cases, it is due to new mutations and, as a result of this, will never be eliminated purely by genetic counselling). It is a relatively rare condition, affecting one in 3,500 live male births. There is currently no cure. However, there is much research into the condition, both into conventional treatment such as breathing support and management of cardiac complications, and also using novel gene therapies.

The identification of the gene in the mid-1980s and the mutations in the gene which lead to a lack of production of dystrophin protein have contributed to an understanding of the underlying cause of Duchenne muscular dystrophy. Dystrophin is essential to the maintenance of healthy, functioning muscle cells. If this protein is absent, the muscle cells will eventually break down and are replaced by connective and fatty tissue, with a loss of muscle function. Now that it is possible to identify the mutation on the X chromosome which causes the condition, it is also possible to offer accurate genetic advice to those females in the families at risk of being a carrier.

Although there is currently no cure for Duchenne muscular dystrophy, over the past few decades, there have been advances in the management of the condition and, consequently, the majority of those affected are now living well into the third and, occasionally, even fourth decades (Eagle et al., 2002).

Effective management involves a multidisciplinary team and includes Physiotherapy, Occupational Therapy, steroid therapy, Orthotics, spinal-fusion surgery, 24-hour postural management, overnight ventilation and cardiology screening. The combination of these interventions has led in some cases to an improved lifespan for those with the condition (Bushby et al., 2005).

The mode of action of steroids is not fully understood. However, they have been found to slow the progression of the condition and delay loss of independent ambulation, possibly through a combination of mechanisms which might include enhancement of myoblast formation, stabilisation of the muscle cell membrane and anti-inflammatory effects leading to reduction in muscle cell necrosis. The spinal fusion procedure uses Luque rods to prevent a kypho-scoliosis from developing and, by maintaining an upright position, is thought to assist lung function and improve posture (Byrne et al., 2003).

Non-invasive ventilatory techniques may be introduced after sleep studies performed by the breathing support team and have improved the quality of life for many young men (Eagle et al., 2002; Kohler et al., 2005).

There are many different strategies currently being investigated with a view to finding an effective gene therapy for Duchenne muscular dystrophy. A review article by Nowak and Davies in 2004 provides an excellent summary of the way in which current research is being targeted.

Until a few years ago, the parents of young boys with a diagnosis of Duchenne muscular dystrophy were told that their sons would probably not live beyond 18 years of age. Such thinking has been restrictive and detrimental to both the parents and their sons in not believing in a future to plan for, which might involve higher education or the pursuit of work, or even independent living. Things are beginning to change now and it is necessary to consider a future for the young man which may also involve sexual relationships and parenting.

This shift in thinking is occurring now, yet services and access to higher education, work skills training and housing have not kept pace. The occupational therapist is in a unique position, working in schools, community paediatric services, in social services and housing, and hospices to make a significant impact for the child and his family, and for the young man in the provision of services and enabling independence.

Many young men are now living with the condition into their twenties and thirties, and this may extend further. These men need to be actively supported to participate fully in all aspects of life. The core skill for occupational therapy is in helping an individual to attain their full potential, which is so important for the boys and young men with Duchenne muscular dystrophy who have so much to gain and also to contribute to the society in which they live. This will involve the development of services and of a change in thinking about Duchenne muscular dystrophy.

# Appendix I  Occupational therapy skills, knowledge base and fields of work

The Occupational Therapist (OT) has a unique role in supporting and working with young men with Duchenne Muscular Dystrophy (DMD), and their families as they can assess and evaluate an individual's physical, psychological and social needs. As the OT's focus is on maximising skills, promoting and enabling independence there is an ongoing role with a young man with DMD. For some children and their parents there is uncertainty of the scope of the OT's role. This is understandable as OTs in Social Services have a different role from Paediatric community therapists and there can be confusion. Part of the OT's role is to help clarify what the different therapy services can offer, so that parents and the young man are clear on the services available to them, and how to access them.

The OT works closely with the Physiotherapist, and with community/Social Services OT colleagues. Working with a child or young adult with DMD there are several skills the OT needs to draw upon. Some of these skills overlap with the Physiotherapist. The list below identifies some of these knowledge and skills areas and is taken from the training curriculum for Occupational Therapists.

These include:

| Fine motor and gross motor skills development | Physical medicine and rehabilitation | Moving and handling training, including bariatrics |
|---|---|---|
| Hand development, including wrist and elbow | Palliative care | Awareness of alternative therapies – including acupressure |
| Contracture management | Mental health – and rehabilitation | Psychological aspects of pain, of loss of function |
| Pain management | Assessment and treatment of children with neuromotor dysfunction | Awareness of feeding and swallowing difficulties |

*Continued*

| | | |
|---|---|---|
| Postural management | Muscular dystrophies | Job opportunities for people with disabilities |
| Continence improvement | Mild and severe learning difficulties | Caring for the caregivers |
| Wheelchair assessment and provision | Assessment and treatment of neuropathies of upper limb | Legal rights and benefits awareress |
| Skin protection and management | Spinal cord injuries | Community care services |
| Relaxation techniques | Epilepsy | Bereavement and loss |
| Management of fatigue | Eating disorders – anorexia | Environmental control systems |
| Housing adaptations | Dyspraxia and perceptuomotor difficulties | Gait patterns and deviations |
| Developmental assessment | Behavioural problems and intervention | Managing transitions from children's to adults' services |
| Strategies for managing spinal fusion | Stress, including anxiety, depression – recognising and problem solving | Orthotic technology – upper and lower limb orthoses including ankle foot orthosis (AFO) |
| Knowledge of current equipment | Cultural awareness | Occupational therapy legal duties and responsibilities |
| Splinting | Orthopaedic conditions | Ergonomics |
| Sensory integration therapy | Neurological impairment assessment and therapy | Ethical and legal issues for therapists |
| Mobility issues, including transport | Paediatric sensorimotor assessment and therapy | Health, diet and exercise |
| Psychodynamic approaches in therapy | Passive and active movements of limbs | Spinal orthotics |
| Clinical seating assessment and provision | Educating other professions | Accessing the educational curriculum |
| Environmental assessments | Assistive technology – for children, for adults | IT equipment – hardware and software |

*Continued*

| Functional assessments | Group dynamics | Management |
|---|---|---|
| Evaluation and therapy in activities of daily living skills | Seating for function and deformity prevention, including different pressure cushions | Knowledge of medical conditions |

It is understood that Occupational Therapists will continue to add to their skills after graduation as continuing professional development.

# Appendix II Occupational therapy seating assessment and recommendation

<u>Child's Name:</u>                          <u>Date of Birth:</u>

<u>Child's Address:</u>                       <u>Date of Assessment:</u>

<u>Therapist:</u>

<u>Chair To Be Used At: Home/School (delete as appropriate)</u>

**Reason for Assessment**

**Physical/Medical Needs**

**Method of Transfer**

**Functional Activity Needs**

       **Home**                     **School**

_____

**Equipment Requirements**

_____

**Current Equipment:** _____

**Assessed in:**

|         | Advantages | Disadvantages |
|---------|------------|---------------|
| Chair 1 |            |               |
| Chair 2 |            |               |

**Recommended Equipment:** _____    **Price:** _____

**Available in Store:**     **Yes** _____  **No** _____  **Don't Know** _____
**(education/health/social work)**

**Therapist's Signature:** _____    **Date:** _____

**Contact Details:** _____

                         _____

*Source*: Adapted from Fife Child Health Occupational Therapy Service – Child Health Manual by Ruth Johnston & Joy Blakeney. Reproduced by permission of Carnegie Clinic.

# Appendix III Occupational therapy seating assessment and recommendation

The following is an example.

**Child's Name:** John F                    **Date of Birth:**

**Child's Address:** 54 High Street,        **Date of Assessment:** 01/05/04

**Therapist:**     Ruth

**Chair To Be Used At: Home/School (delete as appropriate)**

## Reason for Assessment

John has recently moved into the area and his stability and mobility have deteriorated. He now requires some support when sitting at a table for work. He previously sat in a normal school chair with no support.

## Physical/Medical Needs

John's trunk and pelvic control are deteriorating, without support he tends to overbalance to the side at times. This is impeding his upper-limb function. As yet John does not have any contractures.

**Method of Transfer**

When attempting to transfer out of a normal school chair John requires minimal assistance as there are no arms to push up from.

---

**Functional Activity Needs**

John needs to have a chair with increased support to use within the school environment for completing school work. He may also benefit from using this when eating/ drinking.

---

**Equipment Requirements**

– height adjustable to fit under table in class and to be at correct height for good seated position
– arm rests to push up from to enable independence in transfers
– adequate support (lateral/ pelvic)
– adjustable – height, width, etc to accommodate for growth
– easily manoeuvred for use in classroom and dinner hall if necessary

---

**Current Equipment: ____ N/A** _____

**Assessed in:**

|  | Advantages | Disadvantages | Price |
|---|---|---|---|
| **Chair 1** | – adjustable seat height<br>– adjustable arms rest heights<br>– adjustable seat depth | – heavy to manoeuvre/push in/out from desk<br>– seat width not adjustable | |
| **Chair 2** | – reasonably lightweight<br>– adjustable seat width<br>– lateral supports available | – seat depth fixed<br>– not height adjustable<br>– support provided is minimal<br>– fixed armrest height | |

**Recommended Equipment:** Chair 1    **Price:** _____

**Available in Store:**              Yes _____    No  √    Don't Know _____
**(education/health/social work)**

**Therapist's Signature:**                                **Date:**

**Contact Details:**

*Source*: Adapted from Fife Child Health Occupational Therapy Service – Child Health Manual by Ruth Johnston & Joy Blakeney. Reproduced by permission of Carnegie Clinic.

# Appendix IV Occupational therapy seating assessment and recommendation

Child's Name:            Date of Birth:

Child's Address:         Date of Assessment:

Therapist:

Chair To be Used at: Home/School (delete as appropriate)

## Reason for Assessment

e.g.    – New child
        – Outgrown current equipment
        – Condition changed
        – Equipment broken
        – Review

## Physical/Medical Needs

e.g.    – Head and trunk control
        – Scoliosis/spinal jacket
        – Contractures
        – Hip asymmetry/dislocation
        – Surgery
        – Respiratory difficulties
        – Continence
        – Additional medical conditions, e.g. epilepsy
        – Other

**Method of Transfer**

e.g. – Independent
– Assisted
– Hoisted (mobile/tracking)

---

**Functional Activity Needs**

e.g.

| Home | School |
|------|--------|
| – Eating/drinking | – Eating/drinking (snack/lunch) |
| – Play | – Playtime |
| – Communication aid | – Communication aid |
| – Completing homework | – Writing/computer |
| – Toileting (access, e.g. for bottle) | – Toileting (access, e.g. for bottle) |
| – Leisure/relaxing chair (e.g. for change of position from wheelchair) | |

---

**Equipment Requirements**

e.g. – Tray
– Knee block/pommel
– Footplate – type
– Trunk support (pelvic/thoracic)
– Head support
– Straps – groin, vest, harness
– Seat type (flat/ramped)
– Cushion (type – pressure-relieving)
– Forearm support (gutter)
– Size, manoeuvrability
– Adjustability
– Other

---

**Current Equipment:** _____

**Assessed in:**

|  | Advantages | Disadvantages |
|---|---|---|
| Chair 1 |  |  |
| Chair 2 |  |  |

**Recommended Equipment:** _____   **Price:** _____

**Available in Store:**          Yes _____   No _____   Don't Know _____
**(education/health/social work)**

**Therapist's Signature:** _____   **Date:** _____

**Contact Details:** _____

_____

*Source*: Adapted from NHS Fife Child Health Occupational Therapy Service – Child Health Manual by Ruth Johnston & Joy Blakeney. Reproduced by permission of Carnegie Clinic.

# Appendix V  Writing up risk assessments

- These assessments must be completed and updated by moving and handling trainers for staff.
- Make sure that the risk assessment is up-to-date: that there is a current date on the front. The risk assessment must be reviewed on every visit; you need to date and sign *every visit*.
- Use these guidelines to complete a risk assessment. By answering these questions, you will be helped to identify key words to use on the risk assessment.

## Main risk factors

- Does the child/teenager have a level of understanding which is: age appropriate/limited/unknown?
- Is the child/teenager cooperative/uncooperative/unpredictable – if so, why? Re. involuntary movement? Re. behaviour?

## Level of dependence

Totally dependent
Needs assistance to transfer
Some sitting balance
Unable to weight-bear on lower limbs

Minimal active participation
Needs assistance in some situations
Full sitting balance
Able to weight-bear in standing

## Other relevant problems

Epilepsy – type of seizure?
Muscle spasms – type?
Muscle weakness? Where?
Fragility – identify osteoporosis? Dislocated hips?
Pain – explain the nature of pain, when occurs, etc.
Skin condition – sensitivity/any red marked areas?
Sensory loss – explain. Does the child/teenager wear glasses?
History of a fall – has the child/teenager ever fallen or had a negative experience in a hoist or in moving and handling?

Attachments – catheter/NG tube/gastrostomy/other – please identify
Any splints/equipment used by child/teenager? E.g. ankle–foot orthoses/hand
  splints/chest brace/neck support

**Manual handling aids that you need to have ready**

Consider the aids required and identify here. They may include:
Hoist
Sling – size/colour/type – with plastic rods?
Manual handling belt
Sliding sheet – which one?

**Child/young person/family comments/wishes**

- Ask the child/teenager how they like to be moved and handled. Ask them
  to help you fill in the form by giving clear instructions as to how they like
  to be moved. You will need to inform them that if they are too heavy to lift
  manually or unable to transfer safely, then a hoist will be used. This section
  is important.
- Ask the parent if the child/young person is unable to answer.

**Review date/weight**

- Put the date and sign your name on every visit. The risk assessment must
  be current.
- Record the weight of the child/young person.
- Comments – refer to any small change or no change.

Write simply what needs to be done: how, what equipment is needed and how
many people are needed for transfer. Include any specific instructions, e.g.
'Do not hammock sling due to extensor spasms'.

**Re: Outings:** Note down which buggy/wheelchair is needed and straps, as well
as all parts of chair, e.g. footplates, knee blocks, tray, lap strap, bib harness.
For outings, all straps and footplates need to be used. Head rests are essential
for transport.

# Appendix VI  Access checklist

| +/√ | Access checklist | Comments |
|---|---|---|
| | **Access to school** | |
| | Transport | |
| | Escort/assistance | |
| | Storage room | |
| | Dropped kerb | |
| | Sheltered parking/car port | |
| | Access to main door | |
| | Assistance at entrance | |
| | **Mobility to/from classrooms** | |
| | Mode – powered/manual wheelchair | |
| | Walking/walking aids | |
| | Independent with doors | |
| | Outdoor mobility/access to outbuildings | |
| | Assistance/supervision | |
| | **Mobility between floors** | |
| | Lift/stairs | |
| | Independent in lift/supervision | |
| | Space for wheelchair and assistant | |
| | Doors | |
| | **Classroom seating (see separate subjects)** | |
| | Ordinary/supportive/wheelchair | |
| | When to be used? | |
| | Tray or table | |
| | Height-adjustable table | |

*Continued*

| | |
|---|---|
| **Wheelchair** | |
| Manual/powered      indoor/outdoor | |
| When to be used? | |
| Assistance/supervision to transfer | |
| Hoist transfers | |
| Kerb climber/anti-tip | |
| **Standing frame** | |
| See physiotherapist – space/storage, when to be used | |
| **Use of walker** | |
| When to be used | |
| Supervision required? | |
| **Playground** | |
| Access/kerbs | |
| Level/uneven/sloped surfaces | |
| Supervision required? | |
| Wet-weather arrangements | |
| Seating for resting | |
| **Toileting** | |
| Note all bathrooms to be used | |
| Equipment present? | |
| Changing bed | |
| Turning space/space for hoist? | |
| Supervision/assistance | |
| Access toilet and sink | |
| Locker for personal aids required, e.g. urine bottle | |
| **Dining room** | |
| Access – ramp/stairs/level | |
| Seating | |
| Access to food servery | |
| Assistance to carry tray | |
| Assistance/supervision to eat/cut food/drink | |

*Continued*

| | | |
|---|---|---|
| | **Transfers** | |
| | Independent/with minimum assistance | |
| | Transfer board | |
| | Standing hoist | |
| | Mobile hoist with sling | |
| | Tracking hoist with sling | |
| | **Secondary subjects** | |
| | **Craft and design technology** | |
| | Access to room | |
| | Access to workbench/desk | |
| | Seating | |
| | Supervision/assistance | |
| | **Home economics** | |
| | Access to room | |
| | Access to work surface/sink/cooker/microwave | |
| | Seating | |
| | Supervision/assistance | |
| | **Science** | |
| | Access to room | |
| | Access to bench/sink | |
| | Seating | |
| | Supervision/assistance | |
| | **Music/drama** | |
| | Access to room | |
| | Seating | |
| | Access to instruments | |
| | Access to stage area | |
| | Access to sound recording studio | |
| | Supervision/assistance | |

*Continued*

| Languages | |
|---|---|
| Access to language lab | |
| Supervision/assistance | |
| **PE** | |
| Access to department areas | |
| Changing facilities space/plinth/hoist | |
| Showering facilities – level access/chair/bed | |
| Supervision/assistance with changing/showering | |
| Pool access – hoist bed/chair | |
| Recommendations from physiotherapist | |
| **Fire evacuation** | |
| Plan | |
| Safe area? | |
| Evacuation chair/sling/mat | |
| **Other points** | |
| 1 | |
| 2 | |
| 3 | |
| 4 | |

Based on a checklist originally devised by Lynne Rule and Nicola Richardson, Senior Occupational Therapists, NHS Tayside, Armitstead Child Development Centre, Dundee.

# Appendix VII  Housing report

| | | |
|---|---|---|
| Organisation | | |
| Housing Report | | |
| Purpose of Report | | |
| **Client Details** | | |
| Name | | Date of Birth |
| Address | | Telephone |
| Medical Condition | | |
| Mobility | | |
| Care Needs | | |
| Social Network | | |
| Housing Expectations | | |
| **Family Details and Social Network** | | |
| Family Members | | |
| Medical Issues | | |
| Social Network | | |
| Housing Expectations | | |

*Continued*

| Housing Report | | | |
|---|---|---|---|
| Name | | Present Home | |
| | | Proposed Home | |
| | | | |
| House Owner | | | |
| Type and Size | | | |
| Location and Area | | | |
| Car Access | | | |
| Garden | | | |
| Exterior Access | | | |
| Hall | | | |
| Lounge | | | |
| Dinning Room | | | |
| Kitchen | | | |
| Bathroom | | | |
| Client's Bedroom | | | |
| Other Rooms | | | |
| Storage and Heating | | | |
| **Summary** | | | |

*Continued*

| Housing Report | | | |
|---|---|---|---|
| Name | | | |
| **Equipment and Adaptations** | | | |
| Existing Equipment | | | |
| Proposed Equipment | | | |
| Existing Adaptations | | | |
| Proposed Adaptations | | | |
| **Recommendations** | | | |
| | | | |
| **Client's or Parent's Signature** | | **Date** | |
| **Assessor's Signature** | | **Date** | |
| **Cc.** | | | |

# Appendix VIII  Housing assessment

| Organisation | | |
|---|---|---|
| **Housing Assessment** | | |
| Reason for Assessment | | |
| *Client Details* | | |
| Name | | Date of Birth |
| Address | | Telephone |
| Medical Condition | | |
| Mobility | | |
| Care Needs | | |
| Social Network | | |
| Housing Expectations | | |
| *Family Details and Social Network* | | |
| Family Members | | |
| Family Medical Issues | | |
| Social Network Community Integration Informal Carers | | |
| Housing Expectations Acceptable Adaptation Do They Want to Move? | | |

*Continued*

| Housing Assessment | | |
|---|---|---|
| Name | | Present Home |
| | | Proposed Home |

| *House Details* | |
|---|---|
| House Owner | |
| Type and Size | |

| *Area and Location* | |
|---|---|
| Rural or built-up area<br>Flat or hill area<br>Lowered kerbs in area<br>Shops<br>Schools<br>Health centres<br>Hospitals<br>Leisure activities<br>Near family<br>Transport links | |

| *Car Access* | |
|---|---|
| Parking near house<br>Garage<br>Car port suitable height<br>Parking area with WC<br>   transfers area<br>Suitable surface<br>WC access to house from<br>   parking area<br>Disabled parking bay<br>Parking for school bus | |

| *Exterior Access and Garden* | |
|---|---|
| WC access from road to house<br>Number of steps at doors<br>Paths wide enough<br>Surface suitable<br>Ramps suitable gradients and<br>   width<br>Handrails on ramps<br>WC access to garden<br>Safe play area<br>Storage for outdoor equipment<br>Room for extension or<br>   adaptations<br>Can client access and leave<br>   house independently? | |

*Continued*

| Housing Assessment | |
|---|---|
| Name | |

| Hall | |
|---|---|
| Hall 950 mm wide<br>Adequate turning space<br>Fixtures blocking access<br>Threshold hazards<br>Flooring suitable<br>Number of stairs<br>Handrails on stairs<br>Alternative to using stairs,<br>  e.g. lift<br>Lifts accessible and safe<br>Doors wide enough for WC<br>  or hoist<br>Client can open doors<br>  independently<br>Sockets and switches<br>  accessible to client<br>WC storage area with socket<br>  for charging WC<br>Hazards in hall area<br>Can it be adapted to meet<br>  client's needs? | |

| Lounge and Dining Area | |
|---|---|
| Accessible for WC user<br>Enough circulation space<br>Threshold hazards<br>Heating control, sockets and<br>  switches accessible<br>Flooring suitable<br>Client can open windows and<br>  doors<br>View from the window<br>Table a suitable height<br>Hazards<br>Room for postural chair<br>Space for hoist<br>Can they be adapted to meet<br>  client's needs? | |

*Continued*

| Housing Assessment | |
|---|---|
| Name | |
| **Kitchen** | |
| Accessible for WC user<br>Enough circulation space<br>Threshold hazards<br>Sockets and switches accessible<br>Flooring suitable<br>Client can open windows and<br>   doors<br>Cooker controls accessible<br>Cooker and other white goods<br>   accessible<br>Worktops suitable<br>Sink and taps suitable<br>Accessible storage<br>Area to eat meals<br>Hazards<br>Can kitchen be adapted? | |
| **Bathroom** | |
| Accessible for WC user<br>Enough circulation space<br>Threshold hazards<br>Sockets and switches<br>   accessible<br>Flooring suitable<br>Client can open windows and<br>   doors<br>Do fixtures stop access?<br>Enough space and clearance<br>   for hoist/WC/shower chair<br>Is toilet/clos-o-mat suitable?<br>Is toilet paper accessible?<br>Can client flush toilet?<br>Space for transfers<br>Grab rails at toilet<br>Is bath suitable?<br>Is shower suitable?<br>Is shower control accessible?<br>Is washbasin accessible?<br>Are taps suitable?<br>Space for changing table<br>Can bathroom be adapted?<br>Alternative bathroom | |

*Continued*

| Housing Assessment | |
|---|---|
| Name | |
| **Client's Bedroom** | |
| Accessible for WC user<br>Enough circulation space<br>Threshold hazards<br>Heating control, sockets and<br>   switches accessible and<br>   accessible from bed<br>Flooring suitable<br>Client can open windows and<br>   doors<br>Is bed suitable?<br>Is a hoist available?<br>Is there an en-suite bathroom<br>   with hoist?<br>Is there a suitable study<br>   worktop area?<br>Is the bedroom isolated?<br>Is there an alarm?<br>Is there storage for equipment<br>   and possessions?<br>Are environmental controls<br>   needed?<br>Fire alarm<br>Can the bedroom be adapted?<br>Is there an alternative bedroom<br>   that is suitable?<br>Are there enough bedrooms for<br>   the size of the family? | |
| **Other Rooms** | |
| Accessible for WC user<br>Enough circulation space<br>Threshold hazards<br>Heating control, sockets and<br>   switches accessible and<br>   accessible from bed<br>Flooring suitable<br>Client can open windows and<br>   doors | |
| **Storage and Heating** | |
| Equipment storage areas<br>Adequate storage for family<br>   possessions<br>Adequate heating in all rooms<br>Suitable accessible heating<br>Alternative storage areas | |

*Continued*

| Housing Assessment | |
|---|---|
| Name | |
| **Equipment and Adaptations** | |
| Existing Equipment | |
| Proposed Equipment | |
| Existing Adaptations | |
| Proposed Adaptations | |
| Recommendations | |
| | |
| | |
| | |
| | |
| | |
| | |
| | |
| | |
| | |
| Client's or Parent's signature | Date |
| Assessor's Signature | Date |
| Cc. | |

# References

ACT (2003) *A Guide to Effective Care Planning: Assessment of Children with Life-limiting Conditions and their Families*, Bristol, ACT, available online at *www.act.org.uk* (accessed 3/2/07).

Adaptacar (2004) *Information on Wheelchair Accessible Vehicles and Mobility Aids Including Car Seats*, available online at *www.adaptacar.co.uk* (accessed 3/2/07).

Amundson, S. and Weil, M. (2001) 'Prewriting and handwriting skills', in J. Case-Smith (ed.), *Occupational Therapy for Children*, 4th edn, London, Mosby.

Anderson, J., Head, S. I., Rae, C. and Morley, J. W. (2002) 'Brain function in Duchenne muscular dystrophy', *Brain*, **125**, pp. 4–13.

Anemaet, W. K. and Moffa-Trotter, M. E. (2000) *Home Rehabilitation*, St Louis, Mosby.

Audit Commission (1998) *Home Alone: The Role of Housing in Community Care*, London, Audit Commission Publications.

Audit Commission (2007) *Fact Sheet: Help with Transport*, London, available online at *www.audit-commission.gov.uk/disabledchildren/factsheet7.asp* (accessed 12/1/07).

Awaad, T. (2003) 'Culture, cultural competency and occupational therapy: A review of the literature', *British Journal of Occupational Therapy*, **66**(8), pp. 356–63.

Batiiste, L. C. (2005) 'Employees with muscular dystrophy: Job accommodation network', available online at *www.jan.wvu.edu/media/MD* (accessed 3/1/07).

Biggar, D. W. (2006) 'Duchenne muscular dystrophy', *Pediatrics in Review*, **27**, pp. 83–8, American Academy of Pediatrics, available online at *www.pedsinreview.aapublications.org* (accessed 3/2/07).

Birkholtz, M., Aylwin, L. and Harman, R. M. (2004) 'Activity pacing in chronic pain management: One aim, but which method? Part One: Introduction and literature review', *British Journal of Occupational Therapy*, **67**(10), pp. 447–52.

Blom-Cooper, L. (1989) *Occupational Therapy: An Emerging Profession in Health Care*, London, Duckworth.

Bluebond-Langner, M. (2000) *In the Shadow of Illness: Parents and Siblings of the Chronically Ill Child*, New Jersey, Princetown University Press.

Bothwell, J. E., Dooley, J. M., Gordon, K. E., MacAuley, A., Camfield, P. R. and MacSween, J. (2002) 'Duchenne muscular dystrophy: Parental perceptions', *Clinical Pediatrics*, **41**(2), pp. 105–9.

232                                                                    REFERENCES

Brading, J. and Curtis, J. (1996) *Disability Discrimination: A Practical Guide to the New Law*, London, Kogan Page Limited.

Bray, J. and Cooper, J. (2003) 'The contribution to palliative medicine of allied health professions: The contribution of occupational therapy', in Doyle, D., Hanks, G., Cherny, N. and Calman, K. (eds), *Oxford Textbook of Palliative Medicine*, 3rd edn, Oxford, Oxford University Press.

Bresolin, N., Castelli, E., Comi, G. P., Felisari, G., Bardoni, A., Perani, D., Grassi, F., Turconi, A., Mazzucchelli, F. and Gallotti, D. (1994) 'Cognitive impairment in Duchenne muscular dystrophy', *Neuromuscular Disorders*, **4**(4), pp. 359–69, available online at *www.ncbi.nlm.nih.gov* (accessed 15/2/07).

British Red Cross (2007) 'Transport service', available online at *www.redcross.org.uk/localservice.asp?id=2079&cachefixer* (accessed 14/1/07).

Brown, G. (2002) 'Muscular dystrophy', in Turner, A., Foster, M. and Johnson, S. E. (eds), *Occupational Therapy and Physical Dysfunction Principles, Skills & Practice*, 5th edn, Edinburgh, Churchill Livingston.

BRSM – British Society of Rehabilitation Medicine, *Specialized Wheelchair Seating Guidelines*, available online at *www.bsrm.co.uk* (accessed 3/2/07).

Bull, R. (ed.) (1998) *Housing Options for Disabled People*, London, Jessica Kingsley Publishers.

Bumphrey, E. E. (ed.) (1995) *Community Practice: A Text for Occupational Therapists and Others Involved in Community Care*, London, Prentice-Hall.

Bushby, K., Raybould, S., O'Donnell, S. and Steele, J. (2001) 'Social deprivation in Duchenne muscular dystrophy: Population based study', *British Medical Journal*, **323**, pp. 1035–6.

Bushby, K., Bourke, J., Bullock, R., Eagle, M., Gibson, M. and Quinby, J. (2005) 'The multidisciplinary management of Duchenne muscular dystrophy', *Current Paediatrics*, **15**, pp. 292–300.

Bye, R. (1998) 'When clients are dying: Occupational therapists' perspectives', *Occupational Therapy Journal of Research*, **18**(1), pp. 3–24.

Byrne, E., Kornberg, A. J. and Kapsa, R. (2003) 'Duchenne muscular dystrophy: Hopes for the sesquincentenary', *Medical Journal of Australia*, **179**(9), pp. 463–4.

Cadman, D., Rosenbaum, P., Boyle, M. and Oxford, D. R. (1991) 'Children with chronic illness: Family and parent demographic characteristics and psychological adjustment', *Pediatrics*, **87**, pp. 884–9.

Campbell, S. K., Vander Linden, D. W. and Palisano, R. J. (2000) *Physical Therapy for Children*, 2nd edn, Philadephia, W.B. Saunders Company.

Case-Smith, J., Allan, A. S. and Pratt, P. N. (1996) *Occupational Therapy for Children*, St Louis, Mosby.

Catlin, N. and Hoskin, J. (2006) 'Parents' practical strategies for managing behaviour', in PPUK, *Learning and Behaviour Toolkit for Duchenne Muscular Dystrophy*, available online at *www.ppuk.org* (accessed 5/1/07).

Chambers, L. (ed.) (2004) *Inclusive Education for Children with Muscular Dystrophy and Other Neuromuscular Conditions: Guidance for Primary and Secondary Schools*, London, Muscular Dystrophy Campaign, available online at *www.musculardystrophy.org* (accessed 12/6/06).

Chawla, J. C. (1994) 'ABC of Sports Medicine: Sport for people with disability', *BMJ*, **308**, pp. 1500–4.

Chester, H., Freebody, J. and Starkey, S. (researchers) (2001) *Children with Disabilities: Information, Advice, Equipment*, 2nd edn, Oxford, The Disability Information Trust.

Clutton, S., Grisbrooke, J. and Pengelly, S. (2006) *Occupational Therapy in Housing: Building on Firm Foundations*, London, Whurr Publishers.

Cohen, Z. (2003) 'The single assessment process: An opportunity for collaboration or a threat to the profession of occupational therapy?', *The British Journal of Occupational Therapy*, **66**(5), pp. 201–8.

College of Occupational Therapists (2006a) *Risk Management: College of Occupational Therapists Guidance 1*, London, COT.

College of Occupational Therapists (2006b) *Manual Handling: College of Occupational Therapists Guidance 3*, London, COT.

Conneeley, A. L. (1998) 'The impact of the Manual Handling Operations Regulations 1992 on the use of hoists in the home: The patient's perspective', *British Journal of Occupational Therapy*, **61**(1), pp. 17–21.

Connexions (2006) *Parents Carers of Year 9 Students 2006–2007*, Suffolk, DFES Publications.

Cooper, J. and Vernon, S. (1996) *Disability and the Law*, London, Jessica Kingsley Publishers.

Corr, C. A., Nabe, C. M. and Corr, D. M. (1997) *Death and Dying, Life and Living*, 2nd edn, Pacific Grove CA, Pacific Brooks Cole.

Cotton, S., Crowe, S. F. and Voudouris, N. (1998) 'Neurological profile of Duchenne muscular dystrophy', *Child Neuropsychology, Development and Cognition: Section C*, **2**(4), pp. 110–18.

Cotton, S. M., Voudouris, N. J. and Greenwood, K. M. (2001) 'Intelligence and Duchenne muscular dystrophy: Full-scale, verbal, and performance intelligence quotients', *Developmental Medicine and Child Neurology*, **43**, pp. 497–501.

Cotton, S. M., Voudouris, N. J. and Greenwood, K. M. (2005) 'Association between intellectual functioning and age in children and young adults with Duchenne muscular dystrophy: Further results from a meta-analysis', *Dev. Med Child Neurology*, **47**(4), pp. 257–65, available online at *www.ncbi.nlm.nih.gov* (accessed 15/2/07).

Creek, J. (2006) 'A standard terminology for occupational therapy', *British Journal of Occupational Therapy*, **69**(5), pp. 202–8.

Cronin, A. F. (2001) 'Psychosocial and emotional domains', in J. Case-Smith (ed.), *Occupational Therapy for Children*, 4th edn, London, Mosby.

Daoud, A., Dooley, J. M. and Gordon, K. E. (2004) 'Depression in parents of children with Duchenne muscular dystrophy', *Pediatric Neurology*, **31**(1), pp. 16–19.

Dare, A. and O'Donovan, M. (2002) *Good Practice in Caring for Children with Special Needs*, 2nd edn, Cheltenham, Nelson Thornes (Publishers) Ltd.

Darnbrough, A. and Kinrade, D. (1995) *Directory for Disabled People: A Handbook of Information for Everyone Involved in Disability*, 7th edn, London, Prentice Hall, Harvester Wheatsheaf.

Davies, M. (ed.) (2002) *Companion to Social Work*, 2nd edn, Oxford, Blackwell Publishing.

Department of Health (2005) *Hospital Travel Costs Scheme Guidance*, London, available online at *www.dh.gov.uk/assetRoot/04/12/77/39/04127739.pdf* (accessed 13/1/07).

Department of Work and Pensions (2002) *Pathways to Work: Helping People into Employment*, available online at *www.dwp.gov.uk/publications* (accessed 13/1/07).

DfT – Department for Transport (2006) 'The safety of wheelchair occupants in road passenger vehicles: Information on regulatory impact assessment', available online at *www.dft.gov.uk/transportforyou/access/tipws/thesafetyofwheelchairoccupan6168* (accessed 15/2/07).

Dimond, B. (2004*) Legal Aspects of Occupational Therapy*, 2nd edn, Oxford, Blackwell Publishing.

Directgov (2007a) 'How to obtain your free disabled tax disc', available online at *www.direct.gov.uk/en/Motoring/OwningAVehicle/HowToTaxYourVehicle/DG_4022121* (accessed 14/1/07).

Directgov (2007b) 'The Blue Badge Parking Scheme', available online at *www.direct.gov.uk/en/DisabledPeople/MotoringAndTransport/DG_4001061* (accessed 14/1/07).

Disability Rights Commission (2007) 'Employment', available online at *www.drc-gb.org/employment.aspx* (accessed 12/1/07).

Disabled Living Foundation (1994) *Flying High: A Practical Guide to Air Travel for Elderly People and People with Disabilities*, London, Disabled Living Foundation.

Disabled Living Foundation (2005) 'Making a difference: DLF factsheet', DLF, available online at *www.dlf.org.uk* (accessed 17/9/06).

Disabled Living Foundation (2006) 'Choosing a standard self propelled wheelchair factsheet', available online at *www.dlf.org* (accessed 15/2/07).

Disabled Persons Transport Advisory Committee (2001) 'Accessibility specification for small buses designed to carry 9 to 22 passengers (inclusive)', available online at *www.dptac.gov.uk/pubs/smallbus2001/01.htm#1* (accessed 17/1/07).

*Dorlands Medical Dictionary for Health Consumers* (2005) Saunders – an imprint of Elsevier, USA.

Eagle, M. (2002) 'Twenty five years of non-invasive ventilation in Duchenne MD: The Newcastle data', presented on 19/09/02 at the Third Annual Meeting of the Scottish Muscle Network, Glasgow.

Eagle, M., Baudouin, S. V., Chandler, C., Giddings, D. R., Bullock, R. and Bushby, K. (2002) 'Survival in Duchenne muscular dystrophy: Improvements in life expectancy since 1967 and the impact of home nocturnal ventilation', *Neuromuscular Disorders*, **12**, pp. 926–9.

Edmans, J., Champion, A., Hill, L., Ridley, M., Skelly, F., Jackson, T. and Neale, M. (2001) *Occupational Therapy and Stroke*, London, Whurr Publishers.

Emery, A. E. H. (2000) *Muscular Dystrophy: The Facts*, 2nd edn, Oxford, Oxford University Press.

eMove chairs information, available online at *www.asd.co.uk/special_needs/emove/emove/htm* (accessed 21/2/07).

Employment–Solicitors (2007) 'Special needs', available online at *www.Employment-solicitors.co.uk/specialneeds* (accessed 10/1/07).

Enable Together (2007) 'Job Introduction Scheme (JIS)', available online at *www.enabletogether.co.uk/independentliving/employment/jobintroductionscheme.php* (accessed 14/1/07).

Freud, S. (1917) 'Mourning and Melancholia', in *On Metapsychology*, Vol. 11, 1991 edn, London, Penguin.

Goldman, A. (1994) *Care of the Dying Child*, Oxford, Oxford University Press.

Gower's manoeuvre, further information available online at *www.mdausa.org/publications/fa-dmdbmmd-what-html* (accessed 16/09/06).

Greenstreet, W. (2004) 'Why nurses need to understand the principles of bereavement theory', *British Journal of Nursing*, **13**(10), p. 590.

Griffiths, M. (2005) 'Video games and health', *BMJ*, **331**, pp. 122–3.

Guntrip, H. (1992) 'The manic–depressive problem in light of the Shizoid Process', in *Schizoid Phenomena, Object Relations and the Self*, London, Karnac.

Harmer, S. and Bakheit, A. M. O. (1999) 'The benefits of environmental control systems as perceived by disabled users and their carers', *British Journal of Occupational Therapy*, **62**(9), pp. 394–8.

Harper, P. (2002) *Myotonic Dystrophy: The Facts*, Oxford, Oxford University Press.

Harpin, P. (2000) *Adaptations Manual*, London, Muscular Dystrophy Campaign.

Harpin, P. (2003) *Adaptations Manual*, 2nd edn, London, Muscular Dystrophy Campaign, available online at *www.muscular-dystrophy.org/care_support/adaptations/adaptation.html* (accessed 1/10/06).

Harpin, P., Robinson, T. and Tucket, J. (2002) 'Children with Duchenne muscular dystrophy', in Swee Hong, C. and Howard, L. (2002) *Occupational Therapy in Childhood*, London, Whurr Publishers.

Hawkins, R. and Stewart, S. (2002) 'Changing rooms: The impact of adaptations on the meaning of home for a disabled person and the role of occupational therapists in the process', *British Journal of Occupational Therapy*, **65**(2), pp. 81–7.

Healthcare (2004) 'Choosing a wheelchair: Wheelchair seats', information available online at *www.healthcare.uiowa.edu/cdd/multiple/wc/wc_seats.asp*.

Hendry, L. B. and Kloep, M. (2002) *Lifespan Development Resources, Challenges and Risks*, London, Thomson Learning.

Heron, C. (1998) *Working with Carers*, London, Jessica Kingsley Publishers Ltd.

Heywood, F. (2001) *Money Well Spent: The Effectiveness and Value of Housing Adaptations*, Bristol, The Policy Press/Joseph Rowntree Foundation.

Hinton, V. and Cyrulnik, S. (2006) 'Questions and Answers 1.4 in PPUK Learning and Behaviour Toolkit for Duchenne Muscular Dystrophy', available online at *www.ppuk.org* (accessed 5/1/07).

Hinton, V. J., De Vivo, D. C., Nereo, N. E., Goldstein, E. and Stern, Y. (2000) 'Poor verbal working memory across intellectual level in boys with Duchenne muscular dystrophy', *Neurology*, **13;54**(11), pp. 2127–32, available online at *www.ncbi.nlm.nih.gov* (accessed 15/2/07).

Hinton, V. J., Fee, R. J., Goldstein, E. M. and De Vivo, D. C. (2007) 'Verbal and memory skills in males with Duchenne muscular dystrophy', *Developmental Med. Child Neurology*, **49**(2), pp. 123–8, available online at *www.ncbi.nlm.nih.gov* (accessed 15/2/07).

Horner, N. (2003) *What is Social Work? Context and Perspectives*, Exeter, Learning Matters Ltd.

Hyson, L. L. and Sawyer, S. M. (2001) 'Paediatric palliative care: Distinctive needs and emerging issues', *Journal of Paediatric Child Health*, **37**, pp. 323–5.

Jobcentreplus (2007a) *Access to Work*, available online at *www.jobcentreplus.gov.uk/JCP/Customers/Helpfordisabledpeople/Accesstowork/index.html* (accessed 14/1/07).

Jobcentreplus (2007b) *Help for Disabled People*, available online at *www.jobcentreplus.gov.uk/JCP/Customers/Helpfordisabledpeople/index.html* (accessed 14/1/07).

Jones, M. (2003) *Factsheet: Children with Muscular Dystrophy in Mainstream Schools*, London, Muscular Dystrophy Campaign.

Judd, D. (1995) *Give Sorrow Words: Working with a Dying Child*, London, Whurr.

Kapsa, R., Koenberg, A. J. and Byrne, E. (2003) *Neurology Lancet*, 2, pp. 299–310.

Katz, S. (2002) 'When the child's illness is life threatening: Impact on the parents', *Pediatric Nursing*, **28**(5), pp. 453–63.

Kestenbaum, A. (1999) *What Price Independence? Independent Living and People with High Support Needs*, Bristol, The Policy Press.

Kielhofner, G., Butler, J. and Hubbel, W. (2002) *A Model of Human Occupation: Theory and Application*, Baltimore, Lippincott Williams and Wilkins.

Klein, M. (1988) *The Psycho-Analysis of Children*, London, Karnac.

Kohler, M., Clarenbach, C. F., Boni, L., Brack, T., Russi, E. W. and Bloch, K. E. (2005) 'Quality of life, physical disability, and respiratory impairment in Duchenne muscular dystrophy', *American Journal of Respiratory and Critical Care Medicine*, **172**, pp. 1032–6.

Lacy, P. and Ouvry, C. (1998) *People with Profound and Multiple Learning Disabilities: A Collaborative Approach to Meeting Complex Needs*, London, David Fulton Publishers Ltd.

Lanyado, M. and Horne, A. (1999) *The Handbook of Child and Adolescent Psychotherapy*, London, Routledge.

Leeson, J. (1995) 'The child with special needs', in E. E. Bumphrey (ed.), *Community Practice: A Text for Occupational Therapists and Others Involved in Community Care*, London, Prentice-Hall.

Leet, A. I., Dormans, J. P. and Tosi, L. L. (2002) 'Muscles, bones and nerves', in M. D. Batshaw (ed.), *Children with Disabilities*, 5th edn, London, Paul H Brookes Publishing Co.

Likierman, H. and Muter, V. (2005) 'ADHD (attention deficit hyperactivity disorder) and ADD (attention deficit disorder)', available online at *www.netdoctor.co.uk* (accessed 15/2/07).

Lissauer, T. and Clayden, G. (1997) *Illustrated Textbook of Paediatrics*, London, Mosby.

*Longman Modern Dictionary* (1976) London, Longman.

Mandelstam, M. (1997) *Equipment for Older or Disabled People and the Law*, London, Jessica Kingsley Publishers.

Mandelstam, M. (1998) *An A–Z of Community Care Law*, London, Jessica Kingsley Publishers Ltd.

Mandelstam, M. (1999) *Community Care Practice and the Law*, 2nd edn, London, Jessica Kingsley Publishers.

Mandelstam, M. (2001) 'Safe use of disability equipment and manual handling: Legal aspects. Part 1: Disability equipment', *British Journal of Occupational Therapy*, **64**(1), pp. 9–16.

Mannoni, M. (1987) *The Child, his Illness, and the Others*, London, Karnac.

Medical Devices Agency (2001) *Guidance on the 'Safe Transportation of Wheelchairs' Bulletin: Executive Agency of Dept of Health, Social Services and Public Safety*, London, MDA, available online at *www.mhra.gov.uk* (accessed 15/2/07).

Medical Devices Agency (2005) 'Wheelchairs, seating and accessories', available online at *www.mhra.gov.uk* (accessed 12/1/07).

Meggitt, C. (2006) *Child Development*, 2nd edn, London, Heinemann.

Mijovic, A., Turk, J., Hinton, V. and Poysky, J. (2006) 'Behavioural concerns', in *PPUK Learning and Behaviour Toolkit for Duchenne Muscular Dystrophy*, available online at *www.ppuk.org* (accessed 15/2/07).

Motability (2007) 'Motability Home Page', London, available online at *www.motability.co.uk* (accessed 2/2/07).

Murray Parkes, C. M. (1998) *Bereavement: Studies of Grief in Adult Life*, 3rd edn, London, Penguin.

Muscular Dystrophy Association (1998) *Journey of Love: A Parent's Guide to Duchenne Muscular Dystrophy*, Tucson, USA, Muscular Dystrophy Association, available online at *www.mdausa.org/publications/journey/3.html* (accessed 18/8/06).

Muscular Dystrophy Campaign (2004a) *Education Guidelines*, London, Muscular Dystrophy Campaign.

Muscular Dystrophy Campaign (2004b) *Inclusive Education for Children with Muscular Dystrophy and Other Neuromuscular Conditions: Guidance for Primary and Secondary Schools*, London, MDC, available online at *www.muscular-dystrophy.org* (a good resource for schools with overview of all needs).

Muscular Dystrophy Campaign (2006) *Wheelchair Provision for Children and Adults with Muscular Dystrophy and Other Neuromuscular Conditions: Best Practice Guidelines*, London, Muscular Dystrophy Campaign, available online at *www.musculardystrophy.org/information_resources/publications/wheelchair.html* (accessed 1/10/06).

National Rail (2006) 'Rail travel for disabled passengers', available online at *http://nationalrail.co.uk/system/galleries/download/misc/rtdp.pdf* (accessed 12/2/07).

Neuromuscular Centre (2007) 'About us', available online at *www.nmcentre.com/aboutus.htm* (accessed 13/1/07).

Nicolson, R. and Fawcett, A. (2004a) *Dyslexia Early Screening Test*, 2nd edn, London, Hardcourt Assessments.

Nicolson, R. and Fawcett, A. (2004b) *Dyslexia Screening Test – Junior (DST–J)*, 2nd edn, London, Hardcourt Assessments.

Nowak, K. and Davies, K. (2004) 'Duchenne muscular dystrophy and dystrophin: Pathogenesis and opportunities for treatment', *EMBO Rep.*, **5**, pp. 872–6.

Noyes, J. and Lewis, M. (2005) *From Hospital to Home: Guidance on Discharge Management and Community Support for Children Using Long Term Ventilation*, Ilford, Barnardo's.

O'Brien, P. (2003) 'Disabled facilities grants: Are they meeting the assessed needs of children in Northern Ireland', *British Journal of Occupational Therapy*, **66**(6), pp. 277–80.

Office of the Deputy Prime Minister (2002) *Housing Grants*, London, ODPM.

Office of the Deputy Prime Minister (2004) *Delivering Housing Adaptations for Disabled People: A Good Practice Guide*, London, ODPM.

Oldman, C. and Beresford, B. (1998) *Homes Unfit for Children: Housing Disabled Children and their Families*, Bristol, Joseph Rowntree Foundation, Policy Press.

Pain, H., McLellan, L. and Gore, S. (2003) *Choosing Assistive Devices: A Guide for Users and Professionals*, London, Jessica Kingsley Publishers.

Parham, L. D. and Fazio, L. S. (1997) *Play in Occupational Therapy for Children*, St Louis, Mosby.

Parker, J. and Bradley, G. (2004) *Social Work Practice: Assessment, Planning, Intervention and Review*, Exeter, Learning Matters Ltd.

Passmore, A. and French, D. (2003) 'The nature of leisure in adolescence: A focus group study', *British Journal of Occupational Therapy*, **69**(9), pp. 419–26.

Penson, J. and Fisher, R. (eds) (1995) *Palliative Care for People with Cancer*, 2nd edn, London, Arnold.

Piaget, J. (1972) *The Psychology of the Child*, New York, Basic Books.

Picking, C. and Pain, H. (2003) 'Home adaptations: User perspectives on the role of professionals', *British Journal of Occupational Therapy*, **66**(1), pp. 2–8.

PPUK – Parent Project UK (2006) *Learning and Behaviour Toolkit for Duchenne Muscular Dystrophy*, available online at *www.ppuk.org*.

Ricability (2005) 'People lifters', available online at *www.ricability.org.uk/reports/report-mobility/peoplelifters/contents.htm* (accessed 15/1/07).

Rogers, S. L., Gordon, C. Y., Shanzenbacher, K. E. and Case-Smith, J. (2001) 'Common diagnosis in pediatric occupational therapy practice', in J. Case-Smith (ed.), *Occupational Therapy for Children*, 4th edn, London, Mosby.

Saunders, C. (1993) 'Foreword' in Doyle, D., Hanks, G. W. C. and MacDonald, N. (eds), *Oxford Textbook of Palliative Medicine*, Oxford, Oxford University Press.

Scottish Executive (2005) *Supporting Children's Learning: Code of Practice*, Edinburgh, Scottish Executive.

Scottish Homes (1999a) *Adaptations: Good Practice Guide*, Edinburgh, Scottish Homes.

Scottish Homes (1999b) *Access to Housing in Scotland: Rights for Disabled People*, Edinburgh, HomePoint, Scottish Homes.

Shaffer, D. (2002) *Developmental Psychology Childhood and Adolescence*, 6th edn, London, Wadsworth/Thomson Learning Inc.

Shaw, K. L., Hackett, J., Southwood, T. R. and McDonagh, J. E. (2006) 'The prevocational and early employment needs of adolescents with juvenile idiopathic arthritis: The adolescent perspective', *British Journal of Occupational Therapy*, **66**(3), pp. 98–105.

Silcox, L. (2003) *Occupational Therapy & Multiple Sclerosis*, London, Whurr Publishers.

Simonds, A. K. (2001) 'Paediatric non-invasive ventilation', in A. K. Simonds (ed.), *Non-Invasive Respiratory Support: A Practical Handbook*, 2nd edn, London, Arnold/Hodder Headline Group.

Simonds, A. K. (2004) *Factsheet: Making Breathing Easier*, Muscular Dystrophy Campaign, available online at *www.musculardystrophy.org/information_resources/factsheets/medical_issues-factsheets/making_breathing.html* (accessed 13/7/06).

Skelt, A. (1993) *Caring for People with Disabilities*, London, Pitman Publishing.

Skill: National Bureau for Students with Disabilities (2006) *Information Booklet: Making Choices about Leaving School*, available online at *www.skill.org.uk/info/infosheets* (accessed 12/1/07).

Sloper, P. (1996) 'Needs and responses of parents following the diagnosis of childhood cancer', *Child Care, Health and Development*, **22**(3), pp. 187–202.

Sollee, N. D., Latham, E. E., Kindlon, D. J. and Bresnan, M. J. (1985) 'Neuropsychological impairment in Duchenne muscular dystrophy', *Journal of Clinical Exp. Neuropsychology*, **7**(5), pp. 486–96, available online at *www.ncbi.nlm.nih.gov* (accessed 15/2/07).

Souter, J., Hamilton, N., Russell, P., Russell, C., Busby, K., Sloper, P. and Bartlett, K. (2004) 'The Golden Freeway: A preliminary evaluation of a pilot study advancing information technology as a social intervention for boys with Duchenne muscular dystrophy and their families', *Health & Social Care in the Community*, **12**(1), pp. 25–9.

Stalker, K., Jones, C. and Ritchie, P. (1995) *Occupational Therapy: Changing Roles in Community Care?* Edinburgh, The Scottish Office Home and Health Department.

Sterken, D. J. (1996) 'Uncertainty and coping in fathers of children with cancer', *Journal of Pediatric Oncology Nursing*, **132**(2), pp. 81–8.

Stewart, S. and Neyerlin-Beale, J. (2000) 'The impact of community paediatric occupational therapy on children with disabilities and their carers', *British Journal of Occupational Therapy*, **63**(8), pp. 373–9.

Stroebe, M. and Schut, H. (1999) 'The dual process model of coping with bereavement: Rationale and description', *Death Studies*, **23**(3), p. 197.

Sugarman, L. (2001) *Life-Span Development Frameworks, Accounts and Strategies*, 2nd edn, New York, Taylor & Francis Group/Psychology Press Hove.

Tester, C. (2006) 'Occupational therapy in paediatric oncology and palliative care', in J. Cooper (ed.), *Occupational Therapy in Oncology and Palliative Care*, Chichester, Wiley, pp. 107–24.

Tester, C. (2007) 'Bereavement: The pain of loving', in Boog, K. and Tester, C. (eds), *A Practical Guide to Palliative Care: Finding Meaning and Purpose in Life and Death*, London, Elsevier.

Transport Scotland (2007) *The National Entitlement Card*, available online at *www. transportscotland.gov.uk/defaultpage1221cde0.aspx?pageID=241* (accessed 21/2/07).

Turner, A., Foster, M. and Johnson, S. E. (eds) (1996) *Occupational Therapy and Physical Dysfunction*, 4th edn, Edinburgh, Churchill Livingstone.

Turner, A., Foster, M. and Johnson, S. E. (eds) (2002) *Occupational Therapy and Physical Dysfunction*, 5th edn, Edinburgh, Churchill Livingstone.

USAtech (2004) 'United Spinal Association technology guide on wheelchair seat depth', available online at *www.usatechguide.org* (accessed 19/2/07).

Walter, T. (1996) 'A new model of grief: Bereavement and biography', *Mortality*, **1**(1), pp. 7–25.

Waters, B. (2006) *Funding for Disabled Students in Future Education: Skill*, London, The National Bureau for Children with Disabilities, available online at *www.skill. org.uk/info/infosheets/FE%20Fund.doc* (accessed 14/1/07).

WheelchairNet (2006) website providing current information on equipment and complex seating needs, available at *www.wheelchairnet.org* (updated regularly).

Whizzkidz (2003) 'Choosing a manual or sports chair factsheet', available online at *www.whizz-kidz.org.uk* (information on wheelchairs, buggies, cycles and walkers for children with disabilities).

WHO (1998) *Cancer Pain Relief and Palliative Care in Children*, Geneva, WHO.

Wilsdon, J. (1998) 'Muscular dystrophy', in Turner, A., Foster. M. and Johnson, S. (eds), *Occupational Therapy and Physical Dysfunction*, 4th edn, Edinburgh, Churchill Livingstone.

Winnicott, D. W. (1967) *The Child, the Family, and the Outside World*, London, Pelican.

# Bibliography

Baker, S. (2005) *Growing Up, Sex and Relationships: A Booklet to Support Parents of Young Disabled People*, London, Contact a Family.

Baker, S. (2005) *Sex and Relationship Education for Young People with Physical Disabilities: A Booklet for Teachers*, London, Contact a Family.

Case-Smith, J. and Humphry, R. (2001) 'Feeding intervention in occupational therapy for children', in J. Case-Smith (ed.), *Occupational Therapy for Children*, 4th edn, London, Mosby Inc.

Christophers, H. (2005) *Growing Up, Sex and Relationships: A Booklet for Young Disabled People*, London, Contact a Family.

Cohen, H. (1999) *Neuroscience for Rehabilitation*, 2nd edn, London, Lippincott Williams and Wilkins.

Griffin, S. and Price, V. (2000) 'Living with lifting: Mothers' perceptions of lifting and back strain in child care', *Occupational Therapy International*, **7**(1), pp. 1–20.

Ham, R., Aldersea, P. and Porter, D. (1998) *Wheelchair Users and Postural Seating*, New York, Churchill Livingstone.

Kumar, P. J. and Clark, M. L. (1990) *Clinical Medicine*, 2nd edn, Bailliere, Tindall.

Morrow, M., Michael, S. and Clark, J. (2003) 'Ashcraig seating assessment guidance: Duchenne muscular dystrophy', a guide to seating for bio-engineers, physiotherapists, occupational therapists and rehabilitation engineers, and interested parents, available online at *www.gla.ac.uk/muscle/dmd_seating.htm#guide*.

Sales, R. and Utting, J. (2002) 'Manual handling and nursing children', *Paediatric Nursing*, **14**(2), pp. 36–42, Article 760.

## FURTHER READING FOR DEPRESSION AND ANXIETY

Baker, L. L. and Ashbourne, L. L. (2002) *Treating Child and Adolescent Depression: A Handbook for Children's Mental Health Practitioners: Children's Mental Health*, Ontario, Canada, available online at *www.lfcc.onnn.ca/depression_handbook.html*.

Brooks, S. J., Krulewicz, S. P. and Kutcher, S. (2003) 'Kutcher Adolescent Depression Scale: Assessment of its evaluative properties over the course of an 8 week pediatric pharmacotherapy trial', *Journal of Child and Adolescent Psychopharmacology*, **13**(3), pp. 337–49.

Kovacs, M. (1985) 'The Children's Depression Inventory (C.D.I.)', *Psychopharmacology Bulletin*, **21**, pp. 995–8.

Lougher, L. (ed.) (2001) *Occupational Therapy for Child and Adolescent Mental Health*, London, Churchill Livingstone.

National Institute for Clinical Excellence (NICE) has produced guidelines for Depression in Children and Young People (2005), available online at *www.nice.org.uk*.

Dr William Reynolds has produced a Reynolds Child Depression scale (RCD) for under-12-year-olds, and the Reynolds Adolescent Depression Scale –2 (RAD) Reynolds, W. M. (1988), available online at *www.sigmaassessmentsystems.com*.

In the UK, child and adolescent mental health services use different assessment scales, which include: The Hospital Anxiety and Depression Scale (HAD) and the Anxious Thoughts Inventory (AnTI), developed by Adrian Wells. Thanks to the OT Central Scotland CAMHS group for this information.

## FURTHER READING FOR SOCIAL NEEDS

Closs, A. (1998) *The Quality of Life of Children and Young People: Growing Up with Disability*, London, Jessica Kingsley.

Department for Education and Employment (2002) 'Bullying, don't suffer in silence', an anti-bullying pack for schools, available online at *www.dfes.gov.uk/bullying/teachersindex*.

National Children's Bureau (2002) *Making It Work: Removing Disability Discrimination*, available online at *www.ncb-books.org.uk*.

Parent Project Muscular Dystrophy website, with information and resources, including emotional issues, available online at *www.parentprojectmd.org*.

Thompson, C. (1999) *Raising a Child with a Neuromuscular Disorder*, Oxford, Oxford University Press.

## FURTHER RESOURCES

BBC news online, reported 15 November 2006, available online at *www.news.bbc.co.uk*.

*Duchenne Muscular Dystrophy: Research Approaches towards a Cure*, available online at *www.duchenne-research.com*.

Foundation to Eradicate Duchenne Muscular dystrophy, Inc., an American website listing scientific research articles on Duchene muscular dystrophy, available online at *www.duchennemd.org*.

Genetic counselling information, available online at *www.mda.org.au*.

Muscular Dystrophy Campaign, review of research advances in Duchenne muscular dystrophy 2003/4, information available online at *www.muscular-dystrophy.org*.

Parent Project Muscular Dystrophy, information including newsletters and up-to-date information from America, available online at *www.parentprojectmd.org*, including PPMD-produced DVD *Laura's Choice*, reproductive options for carriers of DMD (accessed 21/02/07).

Parent Project Muscular Dystrophy (2007) Information on current research available online at *www.parentprojectmusculardystrophy.org*, click on link for DMD Research (accessed 21/2/07).

Parent Project UK, information available online at *www.ppuk.org*, 'Search for a cure', and Research Archive links (accessed 21/02/07).

Scottish Muscle Network is a point of contact for all professionals working with people with neuromuscular conditions in Scotland; annual update conferences and details can be obtained online at *www.gla.ac.uk*.

Tremblay, J. P. (2004) Quebec research team announces successful trial of Duchenne muscular dystrophy treatment, information available online at *www.cihr-irsc.gc.ca/e/20567.html*.

## SOME WEB ADDRESSES FOR ADD

ADDA Attention Deficit Disorder Association, available online at *www.add.org*, website for adults with ADD and health professionals.

ADDISS, The National Attention Deficit Disorder Information and Support Service – ADHD, Information Services at *www.addiss.co.uk*, *Lessons for Life* booklet, available from this site, providing ways to a child's condition (accessed 15/02/07).

Attention Deficit Disorder, information on articles and aspects of management for parents, available online at *www.ncpamd.com*.

Attention Deficit Disorder (ADD or ADHD) with or without learning difficulties, website for parents, available online at *www.Ld-add.com* (accessed 15/02/07).

Attention Deficit Disorder in the UK, available online at *www.pavilion.co.uk*, providing links with other websites and tips on management (accessed 15/02/07).

Attention Deficit Hyperactivity Disorder information on descriptions, diagnosis, treatment, research and booklets to download, available online at *www.mentalhealth.com* (accessed 15/02/07).

CHADD, Children and Adults with Attention Deficit/Hyperactivity Disorder, available online at *www.chadd.org*, for parents, adults and professionals with training information (USA-based) (accessed 15/02/07).

## DYSPRAXIA ASSESSMENTS

Bundy, A., Lane, S. J., Fisher, A. G. and Murray, E. A. (2002) *Sensory Integration: Theory and Practice*, Philadephia, FA Davis.

Frostig, M., Maslow, P., Lefever, D. W. and Whittlesy, J. R. B. (1963) *Frostig Developmental Test of Visual Perception*, California, Consulting Psychologists Press.

Goodenough, F. F. and Harris, D. (1963) *The Goodenough-Harris Drawing Test*, London, Psychological Corporation.

Henderson, S. E., Sugden, D. and Barnett, A. L. (1992) *Movement Assessment Battery for Children*, London, Psychological Corporation.

## DYSLEXIA

British Dyslexia Association, information and advice; address: 98 London Road, Reading RG1 5AU; helpline telephone number: 0118 966 8271; administration telephone number: 0118 966 2677; information available online at *www.bdadyslexia.org.uk*.

Information on dyslexia services, training, teaching and publications, available online at *www.dyslexia-inst.org.uk.*

Northern Ireland Dyslexia Association, affiliated to the British Dyslexia Association, available online at *www.nida.org.uk.*

*Toe by Toe Multi Sensory Reading Manual for Teachers and Parents,* available online at *www.toe-by-toe.co.uk.*

## SOCIAL SKILLS TRAINING

Baker, J. E. (2003) *Social Skills Training: For Children and Adolescents with Asperger Syndrome and Social–Communication Problems,* London, Jessica Kingsley Publishers.

Social Skill Deficits in Autism Spectrum Disorders, information available online at *www.iidc.indiana.edu/IRCA/SocialLeisure/socialskillstraining.html.*

Spence, S. (1995) *Social Skills Training: Enhancing Social Competence with Children and Adolescents,* Windsor, NFER–Nelson.

Students with Learning Difficulties, social skills training using social stories for training, information available online at *www.udel.edu/bkirby/asperger/socialcaroolgray.html.*

## USEFUL WEBSITES

Backcare: *www.backcare.org.uk*
Calvert Trust: *www.calvert-trust.org.uk*
Children's Wish: *www.childrenswish.org*
Contact a Family: *www.cafamily.org.uk*
Daily Care Ltd: *www.dailycare.co.uk*
DIAL UK: *www.dialuk.info*
Disabled Living Foundation for fact sheets, training packs and courses: *www.dlf.org.uk*
Disabled Persons Transport Advisory Committee: *www.dptac.gov.uk*
Dreams Come True Charity: *www.dctc.org.uk*
Enable: *www.enable.org.uk*
FABB Scotland: *www.fabb.org.uk*
Happy Days Children's Charity: *www.happydayscharity.org.uk*
Holiday Care: *www.holidaycare.org.uk*
Independent Living: *www.independentliving.co.uk*
Make A Wish: *www.make-a-wish.org.uk*
Muscular Dystrophy Campaign: *www.muscular-dystrophy.org*
National Association of Swimming Clubs for people with disabilities: *www.nasch.org.uk*
Outsiders: *www.outsiders.org.uk*
Pocket Guide to Manual Handling: *www.niso.ie/documents/pcketcards.pdf*
Relate: *www.relate.org.uk*
Riding for the Disabled: *www.riding-for-disabled.org.uk*

Royal Society for Disability and Rehabilitation (RADAR): *www.radar.org.uk*
Scottish Disability Sport: *www.scottishdisabilitysport.com*
Scottish Muscle Network: *www.gla.ac.uk/muscle*
Starlight children's foundation: *www.starlight.org.uk*
The Golden Freeway Project: *www.thegoldenfreeway.com*
The Scout Association: *www.scouts.org.uk*
Toilet Aid – Mini Potti: *www.minipotti.co.uk*
Toilet Aid – Uribag: *www.uribag.com/uribag.php*
Tourism for all UK: *www.tourismforall.info*
Wheel Power – British Wheelchair Sport: *www.wheelpower.org.uk*
When You Wish Upon a Star: *www.whenyouwishuponastar.org.uk*

# Index